SKIN ALCHEMY

HOME BASED NATURAL SKIN CARE TECHNIQUES &TIPS

NORA HEDWICK

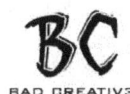

SKIN ALCHEMY

Copyright © 2018 by BadCreative
Art Direction, Cover Design & Typography: Gestvlt

ISBN 9781698617312

All rights reserved.
No part of this book may be reproduced or transmitted in any form or by any means, electronic or mechanical, including photocopying, recording, or by any information storage and retrieval system, without permission in writing from the publisher.

This edition contains the complete text

of the original hardcover edition.
NOT ONE WORD HAS BEEN OMITTED.

A Bad Creative Book / published by
arrangement with the author

BAD CREATIVE PUBLISHING HISTORY
The Simplest Way To Learn Italian published March 2019
The Simplest Way To Learn Spanish, published March 2017

UPCOMING WORKS

Skin Alchemy For Men, 2020
Skin Alchemy For Teens, 2020

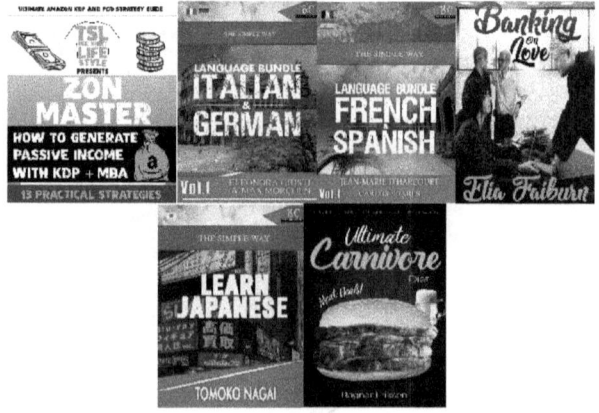

TABLE OF CONTENTS

INTRODUCTION

CHAPTER 1 - THE PHILOSOPHY OF "SKIN FIRST, MAKE-UP SECOND"

CHAPTER 2 - THE FOUR SKIN TYPES AND IDENTIFYING YOURS

CHAPTER 3 - SENSITIVE SKIN AND HOW TO TREAT IT

CHAPTER 4 - WHY REGULAR FACIALS AND A PERSONAL AESTHETICIAN ARE AS IMPORTANT AS GOING TO THE DENTIST

CHAPTER 5 - BAD SKIN CARE HABITS VS HEALTHY SKIN CARE HABITS

CHAPTER 6 - HOW TO BUILD YOUR OWN AT HOME SKIN CARE ROUTINE

CHAPTER 7 - ALL-NATURAL SKIN CARE INGREDIENTS

CHAPTER 8 - MAKING YOUR OWN SKIN CARE PRODUCTS

CONCLUSION

INTRODUCTION

"To be beautiful means to be yourself. You don't need to be accepted by others. You need to accept yourself." I had heard this quote many times before, but it was not until I endeavored to write this book that I truly realized what it meant; or just how true it was.

I am sure that from the time we are very young, many of us are told how pretty everyone thought we were. Moreover, although we accepted these compliments, I am also sure many did not readily consider them to hold any validity. Most likely because of the now overwhelmingly impossible standards of the media watching world, who believe fitting into the mold is what beauty genuinely is.

We are forced to return to our mirrors to figure out just what it is that is wrong with us and what it is that we can do about it — desperately searching for ways to "look good" or "presentable." All the time, not realizing what we were seeking was a way to feel comfortable in our skin.

We start to grow up from being those little girls that everyone called pretty and move over the first threshold into adulthood, our twenties — ultimately becoming increasingly self-conscious and dependent on how others perceive us on the outside. Only feeling confident when someone happens to compliment us, or give us the attention we so desperately need to feel that rush of temporary confidence — returning to our mirrors to figure out why. What was wrong with us that made us so undesirable on the outside?

"What you are inside shows on your face." I am not sure if any of you have heard this saying, but it was not until recently while writing this book in the fact that I came to realize just exactly what those words meant. Moreover, after this epiphany had hit me, I felt the overwhelming need to share it with as many people as I possibly could.

This was also the day that I took another long hard look in the mirror at myself, and I had yet another epiphany. Staring deep into my own eyes, my soul spoke to me. It was not my looks that were the problem. They had never been all along. At that moment, I suddenly somehow understood that what I had previously not liked about my face had nothing to do with my physical features at all. However, it was something else entirely. There was something deep within myself that was being reflected out through my face like some beacon that I had never noticed before now, and it was causing me always to feel those constant feelings of being unattractive, unworthy, unconfident; or just wholly unsettled with myself as a person altogether. I realized right then and there that there were two essential things that I needed to do. Also, I encourage you to do the same.

First and foremost, was to stop spending so much time staring at myself in the mirror. Secondly, probably most crucial of the two was to dig deep, take a look at what was going on inside. Rather than exerting all of my focus on the outside.

I searched all over as well as talked to as many people as I could, whom I believed had more knowledge on this particular subject than I did. Seeing as how they seemed a little more put together as far as their lives were concerned. Whatever, "put together" means, just another one of those general unspecific terms that we as humans like to use to classify other people who seem to be doing life better than we are at the moment.

I had several people recommend meditation, so I gave that a go. I sat quietly, I breathed deeply, quieted my mind, and vocally affirmed my confidence in myself. I was also recommended by several blogs, which I found to be quite ironic, to take a break from all outer distractions and get in touch with myself. However, this method may not necessarily be for everyone right at first. Moreover, I would have to say that it is a clarifying and valuable teaching experience for those of you who feel brave enough to take a break from everything for a couple of days. So I do mean everything. Just forty-eight hours with you, yourself, and you alone. You will find that the solitude will encourage you to reach within yourself. You will desire to meditate, reflect, and be completely one with yourself. It is best to do something like this in an environment that does not permit social interaction, not even fleeting eye contact if you can. Also, no distractions of any kind, such as your phone, television, books, computers, or other digital devices. Just you with yourself.

Will this type of experience be uncomfortable? Unsettling? The short answer is, yes. Some of you may even find it to be quite painful at times. However, I will tell you; it will allow you to bring forth more valuable information about yourself that you would never have unburied otherwise. This experience for me gave birth to one more even more remarkable epiphany. I found that I had suddenly become conscious of just how unnatural I felt in my skin. During this time of deep soul searching and self-acquaintance, I realized that the feeling of being unnatural did not come from not knowing how to be with myself. Instead, it came from the fact that I had honestly forgotten how to be myself. Having forgotten my true identity was the root of all of my gnawing feelings of self-doubt, self-critical thoughts, feeling unattractive, unworthy, or just being overly self-conscious about myself around others. I realized that I had been projecting the persona of someone who was not me, they were only a version of me that I had created to shield myself from what I felt was a harsh world, and people's opinions of how I appeared to them on the outside. The projection became so habitual over the years that it had grown into a "person" of its own. Covering me in a suit of armor that was more like a mask that caused me to forget who I was inside ultimately. The beautiful, confident, capable woman that I was made to be.

Once I was adequately armed with this renewed knowledge of myself, I began my quest to seek my real authenticity and to discover what it was about myself that made me truly beautiful. Not just how I appeared on the outside, but what lay within me.

I gradually began to continue to educate myself and allow life to teach me what things made me happy in my life. After I started this process, I soon discovered that I had found a sort of rhythm, like some deep instinctual music that played inside of me I had never realized before. Even though it had been there the whole time, as it is with all of us, it was miraculous. I had never imagined in my life that I would have my beautiful flow within myself. Also, once I acknowledged its presence, I stayed the course, knowing that it would ultimately lead me to my true authentic self. From there, I knew I would be able to cultivate and rebuild on this new foundation, a strong foundation of realizing who I am. With this knowledge, I gradually began taking my power back. I found that I felt less and less self-conscious around others, not caring whether I fit into their standard of beautiful because I was becoming more and more comfortable with how I fit into my standard of what made me attractive.

A whole new chapter opened in my life. It felt as if I had indeed closed the book on how I had lived my life before. For the first time, I started to think that I was well... that I was beautiful. Not only did I feel this way, but I believed it to be accurate, and it showed. I saw it every time I caught a glimpse of myself in the mirror. Even my husband began to notice it in my body language and demeanor. He began to tell me how I now carried myself differently. It was as if I had more confidence and ease about myself and the world around me. I was not just happy; I was joyful.

Now I would be the first to tell you that this was not a process that happened overnight. Transitions such as this never do. I am also not saying at all that miracles cannot happen, because they do all the time. However, the biggest and most important thing to remember about miracles is that they are achieved through sincere faith and extraordinary effort. So, there were many processes that I used along my quest to find my true beauty. The ones that have assisted me the most and still do, are ones that I continue to apply to keep myself centered. Things such as learning to honor my body.

I can never tell people enough how imperative and essential it is to celebrate the body that you have because it is a gift. We are supernatural beings having a human experience rather than the other way around. So, when they say that your body is a temple, they mean every word. Meaning, you need to treat your body as if it is a temple. Be kind to it. Be sure to thank it every day for all that it does for you. Show it love by listening to and honoring its needs, by doing things like exercising, taking long showers, flossing your teeth, and making sure that you are staying hydrated. Sit down with yourself and make a list of things that you need to do to take better care of yourself so that you can continuously feel happy, healthy, and grounded. Then, make a point to schedule those things into your day. The most important person you can care for is yourself, because the only way that you will be able to serve others best, is when you are at your best yourself. You will also find that it is much easier to feel good about who you are in your skin, when you are taking the time to acknowledge your own needs and make them priorities.

I found that one of the best ways to start this kind of process was by starting with the thing that I wanted to feel most comfortable in, and that was my skin. I found that taking the time to create my at-home skincare routine was not only one of the easiest, but the most significant and most liberating breakthroughs in developing a process of proper healthy self-care. Moreover, this is why I decided to write this book, to share this message with everyone that I possibly can, to show them that they can feel beautiful in their skin even if they need to start just by taking these simple first steps.

Why is proper skincare so important? You ask.

When we have clear, healthy skin, we begin to feel better about ourselves. However, also because our skin, in reality, is one of the main components to preserving our overall health. Your skin is the largest organ of the human body. It covers everything, mostly. So, this is why proper skin care cannot be encouraged enough. It is important because your skin is the most reliable defense against infections that we are exposed to in our everyday lives, often entirely unknowingly. So with proper skincare, it helps to keep this defensive fortress of flesh intact, by preserving the outermost layers of our skin. These layers help to maintain the skin's overall hydration and serve as our primary guardian against the all too often harsh environments we have to live and work in every day. Therefore, doing our best to keep it active and healthy is as important if not even more crucial than keeping our teeth strong and healthy. Also, I know that, for the most part, people see dental care as a pretty high priority. I only wish that they saw just how much proper skincare was in the same category.

Another reason I have written this book, is to spread the message that taking care of the essential component to your entire makeup as a human being is a crucial matter. Not to be taken lightly any longer.

Because this layer of skin serves as such a barrier, it is highly critical that you keep it clean, moist, and healthy. These are the things that keep it secure and able to defend you against free radicals and airborne illness — the first line of defense in your immune system. I am by no means saying that you should use extreme cleaners such as antibacterials, at all times. Harsh cleaners can damage the outer layer of the skin by stripping it of essential lipids and moisture, which it needs to preserve the shield. Often, the use of harsh soaps and cleansers can cause drying and cracks in the skin, which leaves a person even more prone to infection. So it is crucial to make sure that you are using more natural products that are free of heavy scents, perfumes, and chemicals — making sure that the soaps and other cleansers or products that you use on your skin are gentle, as well as creating a habit of using a proper moisturizing treatment every day. Adopting an adequate self-skincare routine into your daily life can help to not only preserve this important protective layer, but also help you to feel better about your overall health in general.

That is what this book is here to teach you. You will not only find out the importance of getting to know your skin by figuring out what kind of skin type you have; you will also learn how to properly care for your skin the way that nature intended. At home. You will equally learn how important it is to find an excellent personal aesthetician as it is to have an excellent personal doctor or dentist. Finally, over the course of this book, you will learn easy techniques and tricks that you can adopt into your daily life at home, to better the health of your skin, and ultimately yourself.

Skin Alchemy   Nora Hedwick

CHAPTER 1

THE PHILOSOPHY OF "SKIN FIRST, MAKE-UP SECOND"

Over the last several thousand years, women all over the world have been chasing the ideal image of glowing skin. The ultimate, flawless, dewy complexion that gives the impression of eternal youth and vibrancy in a person, just by the bright appearance of their skin. A trend that began even before famous ladies such as *Cleopatra*, *Elizabeth the First*, *Audrey Hepburn*, and *Elizabeth Taylor* were at the forefront of what society considered to be the ultimate standard of beauty. The bar for radiant and beautiful skin had been raised ever so high, and seemed to be getting topped every day with excessive media coverage. In recent times, social media filters, Photoshop retouched magazine covers and aggressive advertising tell you that they have the key to what you desire, and in response, the ravenous need to possess this quality has risen to epic proportions.

However, what many women neglect to think about because all these colorful and distracting ads inundate them, is the fact many women before this magnificent obsession used natural products that they created themselves to achieve this effect. Long before women turned to other means of lightening, whitening, and brightening their skin; they were using what nature gave them. As opposed to eventually progressing into ignorance and using things such as harmful chemicals, which created even worse and long-lasting adverse effects, were many times were fatal, and painted their skin with make-up foundations containing elements such as lead and mercury. Then, they'd remove the make-up after wearing it longer than a week with a cocktail that also consisted of substances like mercury and arsenic — seeping into their pores, creating horrible lesions and other unattractive, unsightly markings on their faces, as well as the rest of their skin. Thus, causing them to have to apply even thicker layers of the harmful toxic mixtures to their skin to keep up appearances.

The cosmetics industry has undoubtedly progressed since then, doing their best to try and create products that will give skin this same luminous effect without all of the harmful toxins. However, as of yet this goal has not been completely accomplished, as you will see when reading labels of many of the cosmetic products that you find in either your supermarket, drug store, beauty supply, and even high-end salons or spas that base their reputations on their practices being safe for your skin. Many of these products are still known to be harsh enough to cause irreversible oxidation, erosion, and tarnishing of what would generally be considered heavy metals. Now think about that for just a moment. You are putting something on your face that can eat metal, and you wear this on your face for several hours a day. Sometimes not even bothering to take it off before you go to bed at night.

Furthermore, I would like to state that when it comes to pursuing that perfect, flawless glowing face of radiant make-up; it is false advertising. When we are watching television, flipping through magazines, or merely going through the cosmetics section of a store; we are exposed to ads for these products. Please keep that in mind when you are viewing these things, and you see the model's perfect skin in the commercial, and it makes you want to purchase this product. Understand this is precisely the point. Don't be fooled as we all often are by a good ad campaign. These models who appear flawless and seemingly perfect, are worked on for hours ahead of time by a team of stylists and professionals. All are endeavoring to get her look to be precisely right, and help her look more appealing for the ad. Thus, making the product seem more attractive because it appears to be doing its job. Graphic artists also come in during post-production and use digital airbrushing techniques and bright lighting and filters to remove any other pimples, moles, and freckles which an overly judgmental, and self-critical society sees as imperfections. There are also lighting experts and gaffers being paid to do the job of highlighting only all of her best features, and they do just that. These are the only things that you see. A person who has been heavily painted, airbrushed, filtered, and lighted for the benefit of selling the product to you, the consumer. They are cleverly neglecting to tell you that results may vary from person to person, and there is no way on God's green earth that you will ever look as ideal as the model in the photo or commercial. Unless, of course, you somehow find yourself filming an ad for a cosmetic. It is as simple as that.

I hate to burst your bubble, but this is the truth. Yes, you can buy the product, and it may work relatively to your satisfaction. However, please, stop setting yourself up for disappointment by buying into the fantasy that is the cosmetic advertising industry. Even though many stores such as CVS have begun to pledge to move toward a more non-retouched photo look for their store displays and ad campaigns. We cannot count on everyone to follow suit. So, you will not find out how the make-up appears indeed until you try it yourself.

I am in no way one of those people who run around chanting that make-up is evil, and it's trying to kill you. Nor am I one of those people, who say that you should give it up altogether. I would be one of the first to agree that there is nothing like the feeling of seeing yourself in a flawless face of make-up, and finding a foundation that suits your skin's texture and color, as well as finding complementary shades of blush and eyeshadow that ultimately complete the look. Along with some finishing touches like a subtle highlighter to give you that radiant, fairy childlike glow that everyone is after. There is absolutely nothing wrong with this. However, I am urging you to be more conscientious about your make-up choices, as well as using cosmetics responsibly when it comes to caring for your skin and its long-term health. Which in the long run, ultimately affects your overall health as well.

In order to find the balance between keeping your own skin radiant and healthy, so that you are able to keep the canvas on which you apply your makeup clean and healthy; I am going to tell you that the first and most important action you should take is to start reading the labels of the cosmetic products that you purchase for yourself, as well as asking make-up artists and aestheticians about the products they are using on you, if you are getting a facial or a make-over at a salon or spa. Don't be afraid to educate yourself. Ask questions. Knowledge is power. Also, do not be scared to speak up. If you know that there is a specific ingredient that you have noticed to cause you any irritation or adverse reaction of any kind in your cosmetic products, be sure to tell the person who is working on your face that this is so. It will save much pain, irritation, and heartbreak for you in the future. So, for the most part, those people who are hopefully well educated in their profession and care about the well-being of their customers will be understanding.

When it comes to elite natural skin care, certain parameters have to be observed in your quest for perfect, flawless skin. We'll kick things off from the cosmetic side of things.

VET YOUR COSMETICS

As far as choosing cosmetics is concerned, what you need to be looking for when you are deciding to make the jump towards a healthier route for your skin is this; be sure to select products that have words such as "Non-acne-genic" or "Non-comedogenic" on the labels. These will be less likely to put you at risk for getting acne flare-ups from wearing them for prolonged periods. I am not saying this utterly eradicates any risk of occurrence in the product. It only means it is less likely to occur in products with these words on the label. They are less likely to clog your pores as a product without these words on the label. You still have to make sure that you are cleaning your face, regardless of whether it says it is less likely to clog your pores or not; this is just common sense and an excellent habit to institute. Which we will talk more about later.

It would help you to look for make-up that is water-based as opposed to being made with an oil base, as this is also less likely to cause pore-clogging and breakouts. Especially if you already have oily or combination skin. Not to mention, it gives more of a matte finish that mimics the appearance of a naturally flawless complexion, rather than appearing shiny and causing your pores to grow in size because they can't breathe. Again, I cannot reiterate this enough; your skin is an organ. Which do you think would work better for you if you were walking around in the desert? Offering you a glass of water, or a glass of oil, I think the answer to which would serve you better in that situation is pretty clear without having to explain too much. The same is true for your skin. So always go with a water base rather than oil. You and your skin need hydration and air to live.

TAKE THE MASK OFF!

Stop wearing your make-up to bed! I know, I know, it can be very tempting to go straight to bed, for whatever excuse you can come up with, without washing the make-up off of your face first. However, leaving the make-up that has been sitting on your face for the better part of probably the last eight to twelve hours or so will ultimately clog your pores and cause acne break out. So, make an effort to wash the make-up from your face before you go to bed with a gentle cleanser or make-up remover, using a soft washcloth or cotton pads. If you use any topical acne medication, now would be the best time to apply it; while your face is clean, and you won't be applying any make-up for the next several hours.

Another thing to be aware of is expiration dates. Many people will tell you, "Oh, well, a lot of these products have expiration dates; even though they don't need them..." Not true! The expiration dates are on there for a reason. The same reason why there are expiration dates on food. Because, after a certain amount of time, especially with all-natural products that do not contain copious amounts of harmful preservatives, they expire.

Most of the time, eye make-up is the first to go, because it has the shortest shelf life of many cosmetic products. So, say, for instance, you have a tube of mascara that is about four months old. It would be best if you replaced it with a fresh vial. Also, be aware that you do not share make-up or make-up tools with anyone. I don't care if they are your sister, or your mom, your identical twin...whoever. Please don't do it! Our skin protects us from harmful bacteria that can cause infections and illnesses, and (much like our mouth) how it accomplishes this is that it produces an even more vicious bacteria that it secretes as a layer, onto the top layer of our skin.

It is imperative to note that no two person's DNA are alike; the reason to keep this in mind is that once the bacteria from say your mom or whoever is transferred onto a mascara brush, and you borrow the mascara and use the same brush, even though you came out of your mother and you are made up of a good chunk of her DNA, yours is still different. This means that the bacteria from her dead skin and eyelash hair follicles that made it onto that brush are going to mutate when it comes into contact with the bacteria near your eye. Very possibly causing something as minor as an eye irritation, or something a little worse like a sty, or in an even worst-case scenario, pink eye. All this from sharing a make-up utensil that someone else used, who may or may not have had an infection at any time recently. Also, you don't know if they were studious and responsible enough to throw out the tube of mascara after having had an infection. It's best to throw out make-up that touched any part of your face during the course of an illness. The reason for this is because the germs from the disease are carried out through your pores by the bacteria, sweat, and other such things; leaving you at risk to catch the same bug you had or come down with an even worse secondary infection. So, when in doubt, throw it out!

While we are on the subject of make-up, never do things such as apply eye make-up to the inside of your lid, because this may irritate your eye. Especially if you wear contacts, this can be a complete disaster. Another problematic thing that I see is women trying to apply their make-up while they are driving or riding somewhere. Please refrain from trying to put on make-up in a car or on a bus, as a bump or an unexpected swerve can cause you to scratch your eye or get make-up and other germs in it.

CURB HARMFUL SKIN HABITS

Other such things that can put a crimp in your walk towards having the perfect skin, are continuing with habits that are harmful to your skin. Habits that cause you to have acne breakouts, redness, and scarring. These include practices such as popping your pimples, or generally just picking at your skin. Do not do this. It does not help you to pop your pimples and other offending break outs such as blackheads with your fingers, which are covered in bacteria and germs from you touching various things; then transferring that dirt and grime into your now open wounds with hands that are not clean. You'd be smearing dirt, viruses, dead skin, and bacteria all over your face and making matters much worse, inevitably causing an even bigger break out that you can't seem to explain. Also, keep harsh products such as hairsprays and gels away from your face. They will clog your pores trapping more dirt, grime, and bacteria in them; with some of them also causing breakouts and redness. Avoid wearing tight headbands and wool hats that can irritate your skin. For those of you who smoke out there, please stop it. Smoking is one of the most significant contributors to premature aging of the skin, not to mention it can cause it to be sallow and dry.

The best way to move towards having a good face of radiant, natural skin, is by implementing healthier habits in your life. It will not only help your skin, but will also contribute to the betterment of your general health. Treat your body with the love and respect that it deserves, and that you deserve.

EAT SMARTER

Begin to keep your skin healthy by eating smarter. Fill your plate with veggies, fruits, and whole grains; all things which help to lower your cortisol, which is a stress hormone. They can also boost your vitamin C levels and help you to produce more collagen, which helps not only with keeping down pimples, but it also helps to keep signs of aging at bay longer. Choose leaner proteins such as chicken, fish, lean red meats,(*See the Ultimate Carnivore Diet by Ragnar Eriksen*) beans, and eggs, as these will help to reduce inflammation and fluid retention, giving your skin back its elasticity and helping you not to look quite so puffy when you wake up in the morning. Avoid foods that are high in bad cholesterol, trans fats, processed white sugars, and excessive amounts of processed salt. These also cause inflammation and fluid retention, not to mention that they cause you to be tired longer and crash faster. The continual stress they put on your body, will often appear as wrinkles, dryness, redness, and splotchy-ness on your skin. For a more in-depth look at this particular point, see my book about how to eat your way to clearer skin and better health.

Now that you have gotten this part of the process under your belt, here are a few other crucial points to consider when it comes to setting the foundation for a pallet of radiant, beautiful natural skin.

STOP SLEEPING ON SLEEP

If you are not getting enough sleep, this is something that you need to work on right away. It is one of the most crucial things required to give your skin back that healthy glow. It is vital to your body's overall function that you get at least 6-8 hours of sleep every day. It will soothe your skin and prevent it from looking dull, puffy, and tired.

HYDRATION

Another point that I cannot stress enough is hydration, hydration, hydration! The human body is made up of seventy-five percent water. The right amount of this water lives in your skin. However, as we all know, water tends to evaporate. Whether it be through heat or exertion, you lose gallons of water a day as you go about your daily tasks. I would honestly have to say that water is most definitely one of the biggest keys to curing and preventing the majority of, if not all, of your skin related issues. The more water you consume, the better it is for your skin. So, it is essential that you take in at least two gallons of water per day. Not only will this help your skin, but it will also help the overall function of the rest of your body; such as your energy levels, your muscles, and your joints, and your mind will be more precise.

When pursuing that flawless face, you need to keep in mind that make-up can only make you look as good as the quality of the skin upon which it is applied. So, implementing proper skincare regiments is a must, if this is a goal that you want to accomplish. If you are looking specifically to bring a youthful, vibrant glow back to your skin, speak with your aesthetician about products that are safe for treating dull skin and bringing the light back into your particular skin type. Also, do your best to indulge in healthy skincare practices daily, as a maintenance measure in between visits, and without fail.

You can also opt for a fruit-based mask when you go for your next facial or make one yourself at home, to give your skin a brighter, more illuminated look. Fruits such as papaya, oranges, and grapefruits are very well known for their healing properties and the ability to rejuvenate your skin. They are full of nutrients, minerals, and enzymes; to assist in replenishing your skin cells, and making your skin glow. As mentioned earlier, they are packed full of vitamin C and encourage the production of collagen by reducing the presence of cortisol. They also change the PH in your skin which shrinks your pores, tightens your skin, and makes it difficult for dirt to live on your face for very long. You will see fewer pimples and blackheads populating your face if you go with this method, so I highly recommend opting for fruit-based masks such as these.

As we age, with every passing day, your skin is going to lose its elasticity and original glow. A fact of nature that is inevitable. Not wholly unavoidable however, as long as you have the right tools at your disposal. One of the most efficient ways that I have found to rekindle the glow in someone's skin is by applying specific serums and lotions. Serums especially are also of crucial importance to your skin's health. When you directly use a few drops of serum on your face before bed, it can make all the difference in the world to how your skin appears in the morning. Best practice is to include at least one serum in your daily skincare routine at all times.

Now, we have covered some basic principles of what you require in order to set up the right foundation for your skin. But before you go out and choose your perfect foundation, I think it is time we move onto one of the most critical areas of starting your journey to a healthy canvas for your make-up; as well as understanding how to prevent minor and significant issues with your skin in the future. Specifically, getting to understand your skin type and how to care for it properly.

CHAPTER 2

THE FOUR SKIN TYPES AND IDENTIFYING YOURS

There are four basic skin types of healthy skin; normal, dry, oily, and combination skin. Each unique skin type is subject to genetics. However, the condition of our skin can vary significantly according to many various internal and external factors that we subject ourselves to on the daily.

If you need help in identifying your particular skin type, there is a simple skin test that you can do that is a beneficial tool. However, if you find that you need further assistance or advice on how to best care for your skin type, I highly suggest that you get in touch with a reputable dermatologist, pharmacist, or aesthetician. I believe though, that a person must invest in taking the time to nail down a personal and trustworthy dermatologist and aesthetician, regardless of whether you feel you need advice or not. Just as you put the time and investment into having an excellent dentist and primary care physician, or specialist if you have some pre-existing condition that needs attending to, it is just as important to treat your skin's health with the same amount of reverence and priority as the rest of your health. Because, your skin is where the preservation of your overall health begins. As stated before, your skin is an organ, and because it is porous, it is a gateway into your body for all sorts of toxins and contagions. It behaves like a barrier between you and the rest of the world; which is full of harmful elements. So, to keep this barrier healthy, it must be well cared for, and understanding better what type of skin you have is the first step in being able to care for it properly yourself.

NORMAL SKIN

The "Normal" skin type is often and widely referred to as well-balanced skin. Because, honestly, what is normal? Another unspecific term that people use to classify something they feel someone has that is better than theirs. So, I prefer to use the word well-balanced, simply because this does describe this skin type best. Another reason is that balanced skin is neither too dry nor too 'wet,' or in other terms, oily. When you travel further into the more scientific parts of this kind of research, you will find that well-balanced skin is more explicitly referred to as eudermic. The T-zone area (forehead, chin, and nose) of the individual with this skin type may tend to be a bit oily at times, but the overall sebum and moisture are balanced. Therefore, the skin is considered to neither be too oily or too dry. This kind of surface is identified by the telltale signs of little to no imperfections, no severe sensitivities to speak of, and this person is not readily prone to any adverse sensitivities in regards to their skin. Other signs are, barely visible or very fine pores, a naturally radiant complexion, good blood circulation, a smooth, soft, and even velvety texture, as well as a fresh, and sometimes what is considered a rosy color uniform transparency. If you can identify with any of these traits when it comes to observing your skin; then most likely, you have a well-balanced or eudermic skin type. Something to keep in mind however, is that as a person ages, "normal" fair skin can tend to more often than not become dryer over time. So, making sure that you are taking the time to hydrate yourself as well as your skin is a must, even if you still consider yourself to be a relatively young person. The factor of dehydration plays a considerable role in age-induced dryness. So again, to ward off the signs that Father Time is catching up with you, by all means, keep yourself, all of yourself, appropriately hydrated.

DRY SKIN

The Dry skin type is usually a category that is used to classify and describe skin that tends to produce less sebum than well-balanced skin. Also, as a result of this lack of sebum, the skin lacks the lipids that it needs to help the skin properly retain the moisture that is required for it to stay well balanced, as well as preserve the protective shield against external adverse influences. It ultimately leads to an impaired barrier function, causing dry skin. Dry skin, otherwise classified as Xerosis, exists in varying levels of severity and in sometimes varied and differing forms that are not always very clear or distinguishable — making it difficult to diagnose it accurately at times and causing many dermatologists and aestheticians to tell the individual that they have sensitive skin. In many cases, having dry skin can put you at a higher risk to have sensitive skin, due to its lowered defenses. However, we will talk more about this later. Before that, here are some info about dry skin.

- Skin tends to get much dryer as it ages.
- Significantly more of the female population suffers from dry skin than their male counterparts.
- Problems that are related to dry skin, such as the sudden appearance of sensitivities that were not previously there, are a common complaint of many of the world's population in general and account for over forty percent of visits to dermatologists alone.
- Since our body produces and retains less and less water as we age, extremely dry skin is most commonly found in those who are elderly. Alternatively, on people who work with their hands very frequently, thus making their hands severely dehydrated and leading to such problems as eczema and psoriasis over time, if these issues continue.

So, what are the leading causes of dry skin? Allow me to explain.

Skin's moisture depends significantly on its supply of water in the deeper skin layers and on perspiration. Hence, I will mention this once again. Stay hydrated. Your skin is continually losing water through various methods. One leading cause is perspiration; even though this temporarily provides some hydration, the act of sweating is active water loss from the glands in your skin; which is caused by heat, stress, and physical activity. Another primary cause of water loss from your skin is **Trans-epidermal water loss** or TEWL. It is merely the natural, passive way in which skin diffuses about half a liter of water a day from the deeper layers of your skin.

Dry skin however, is caused by a lack of natural moisturizing factors. Especially, urea, amino acids, and lactic acid that all help to bind in water. Epidermal lipids such as ceramides, fatty acids, and cholesterol are among the moisturizers which your skin barrier needs to function healthily. A lack of these essential factors results in the risk of the skin's barrier function being compromised, and ultimately causing you to have dry skin.

As I mentioned earlier, diagnosing dry skin is difficult at times. The reason for this is that there are varying levels and subtypes of dry skin within the category of what classifies as a dry skin type. Dry skin ranges from the skin that can be just a little bit drier than usual, through to Very Dry skin, and then, of course, there is Extremely Dry skin. These differences can many times be distinguished between by separating them into levels.

DRY SKIN

At first you have just Dry Skin, which is mildly dry skin. It can feel tight, slightly brittle, rough, ashy, and look altogether dull. The skin elasticity is also low, often causes the individual to look just slightly a bit older or more tired.

VERY DRY SKIN

If the dryness goes untreated at the first signs of the first level, then it can progress to this slightly more serious level. It's often identified by mild scaling, patches of flakiness, a rough, blotchy appearance; and even sometimes worsening things with the appearance of premature aging. There will also be present, a feeling of tightness to the skin, as well as itchiness. This level of dry skin also is at risk of being more sensitive to irritation, redness, and higher chances of infections. Often, said infections are responsible for moving the skin into the position of our last classification.

EXTREMELY DRY SKIN

Extremely Dry Skin will appear throughout some regions of the body, more specifically the hands, feet, elbows, and knees; as these are places that are devoid of water in the first place, compared the rest of your body. This makes them more prone to signs of roughness and chapping, with a risk or tendency to form cracks (or Rhagades), calluses, and scales. At this stage it becomes clear to you that if you have dehydrated skin, there will be frequent and more intense itching present.

NATURE AND CAUSES OF DRY SKIN

Dry skin is often pinpointed by the appearance of nearly invisible pores, a dull, rough complexion, red patches, skin with low elasticity, and more visible lines and wrinkles. Skin dryness is what causes wrinkles and more pronounced lines to be more prominent in older women. Also worthy of note is the fact that your skin may exhibit signs of cracking, peeling, or become itchier and more irritated or inflamed, seemingly for no reason. If it is parched, it can even become rough and scaly, particularly on the backs of your hands, arms, and legs.

These conditions can be made worse or even caused by factors such as genetics, aging, and hormonal changes. The weather, such as the sun, wind, or even colder temperatures can equally serve as a drying factor. Also, exposure to UV light radiation from tanning beds, indoor heating, long hot baths, and showers; as well as ingredients in soaps, cosmetics, or cleansers, can significantly contribute to acute skin dryness. Finally, different prescription medications which many of us are required to take for other issues, can come with the side effect of severely dry skin.

DRY SKIN MANAGEMENT AND REMEDIES

If you find yourself suffering from any of the symptoms that I have listed above in this portion of the chapter, here are some practical measures that you can take to help manage your dry skin better.

- It will help if you take shorter showers and baths, no more than once a day. Opt to use milder or gentler soaps and cleansers, and at all costs, avoid deodorant soaps. Especially ones that say they will help you to perspire less.
- Do not scrub while bathing or drying. Patting or air drying is best if you have dry skin.
- Liberally apply a rich, deep penetrating moisturizer directly after bathing. Ointments and creams may tend to work better than lotion on dry skin, but I tend to find these to be a lot messier. Feel free to reapply as much as needed throughout the day.
- Use a humidifier, and do not allow indoor temperatures to become too hot.
- Make a point to wear gloves when using cleaning agents, solvents, or other household cleaning products or detergents; as these tend to be made with harsh chemicals and astringents that will quickly suck all of the excess moisture out of anything. Especially your skin.

OILY SKIN

Just as dry skin is classified as skin that produces less sebum than well balanced, or "normal" skin, the oily skin type is often identified by the fact that it has a heightened amount of sebum production than the other two. What is sebum you ask? Sebum is the oily substance that is produced by our body's sebaceous glands to keep our hair and skin supple. When there is an excess of this secretion, the overproduction is then referred to as **seborrhea**. A condition often typified by more acne or blemish-prone skin.

The causes for this overproduction of sebum typically are, of course, your genetics, hormonal changes and imbalances such as puberty or pregnancy, prescription medications with side effects that may cause increased sebum, stress, and last but not least comedogenic cosmetic products. These are products that cause irritation and clogging of your pores.

The signs of such things can identify this particular skin type as enlarged pores, dull or shiny, often thick looking complexion, a population of pimples, blackheads, or other blemishes. Oily skin can also be characterized by the appearance of paler skin and lessened visibility of blood vessels under the skin.

This increased level of excess skin barrier causes the skin to be exponentially oily, and makes the skin more prone to such things as a significant number of comedones appearing on the face, and frequently on the neck, shoulders, back, and chest of the individual as well. Comedones are a long term that is used to identify or classify such things as blackheads and whiteheads, which are the symptoms and byproduct of acne (A condition that is more often caused by an increased level of sebum secretion by the skin).

In moderate and severe cases, papules (small bumps with no visible black or white head), and pustules (medium-sized bumps with a noticeable yellow or white dot at the center of the breakout) make an appearance on the skin, and over a short amount of time become red and inflamed.

ACNE

More often than not, acne is classified as an inflammatory disease, because inflammation is present at every stage of its inception. Several myths are often associated with those who have acne and as to the reason why they have it. For instance, people that have more blemishes on their skin than others are less hygienic than everyone else. It is blatantly, not true. And also, most would be quick to say that acne is directly caused by an excess of oil or sebum on the skin, this is not always the case. There are many other factors to take into consideration, concerning why a person is more likely to be prone to having acne than others. They include:

GENES

A few key elements that medical professionals have been able to pin down are things such as your genes. Genetics determines your skin type, and many of us have more reactive skin at risk for inflammation, blemishes, and acne than other people around us. If both your parents suffered from acne any time in their life, then you are at a higher risk of developing the condition. It's just a fact.

HORMONES

Your hormones are another factor. Acne is often categorized as a hormonal disease, or rather the symptom of an extreme hormonal surge or imbalance. Your hormones are the ones responsible for the development of your sebaceous glands. Hence, they stimulate sebum production in those glands. This ties into the fact that overproduction of this particular secretion is one of the telltale signs that a person is more prone to blemishes, aka Oily Skin. Though this is not the only cause, it is quite a hefty contributor.

The increase in hormones during puberty is the most common reason why acne is more common in adolescent members of society. However, hormones continue to affect men and women quite differently at various stages of their life. There are changes in hormonal levels during a woman's menstrual cycle to consider, which more often than not causes a flare-up, most typically for women in their twenties and thirties.

PRESCRIPTION MEDICATION

I know I mentioned these to be a contributing factor for why your skin is behaving the way it is, along with a couple of the others on the list. However, people do not take the time to consider just how much prescription medication has an effect on your skin and how it changes over time. Some medicines for instance, steroids and even some anti-depressants like lithium, will cause acne flare-ups.

YOUR DIET

There is quite a bit of evidence to support the correspondence between a person's diet and how much or how little they are prone to conditions such as acne. A menu that is high glycemic, and features many dairy products, may not only trigger, but also continuously exacerbate an individual's acne problem.

STRESS

Stress is another factor. Stress causes an imbalance in your hormones because when you stress, your body is producing more cortisol and less collagen — also depleting your body's supply of things such as Vitamin C, D, and E. Which in turn stimulates an increased production of sebum that will also bring about acne.

SMOKING

This is definitely in the top five for sure, as far as causes of multiple types of skin aggravations - everything from skin dryness and premature aging, to depletion of oxygen and hydration, and causing oxidative stress on the body. Smoking alters your sebum PH and composition, creating an at risk for acne zone, namely your skin.

HARSH LIPIDS AND CLEANSERS

Improper skincare such as the prolonged use of harsh antibacterial or anti-fungal soap-based cleansers, and water that is entirely too hot not only can, but will also disrupt your skin's natural balance and cause such symptoms as acne.

OTHER BODILY PROCESSES

The excess of sebum on the skin's surface often interferes with the natural processes that the skin uses to rid itself of dead skin cells — a process known as desquamation. In other cases, the makeup of the sebum lipids that build up in the sebaceous glands also can cause micro-inflammations.
Acne can also be triggered by other conditions such as Hyperkeratosis, which is an abnormal thickening of the outer layer of your skin caused by an excess of cell production, also triggered by sudden hormonal changes and dry desquamation of cells. These dead cells then form into blockages that plug up the sebaceous glands, producing sebum to build up in the follicle wall, making it bulge; which creates comedones — a byproduct symptom of the acne condition.

Bacteria also play a role here. I don't know if you recall that I mentioned earlier in the book, there are harmful bacteria that live in the barrier that is over your skin, protecting it from outside infections and contagions. Just like the bacteria that resides in your mouth, it has adapted itself to be more vicious than what it fears will attack you, to make its protection of your health more effectively. The bacteria that exist typically quite harmlessly on the surface of your skin are known as Propinionbacterium acnes (or P. Acnes). However, harmless it may be for everyone else with relatively healthier skin and healthier habits, for people with more acne-prone skin; it can cause them to be more sensitive to themselves. Thus, triggering some inflammation. Excessive sebum production also creates an environment that helps P. acnes to grow and thrive. It begins to colonize in the ducts of the now plugged sebaceous glands causing even further inflammation and ultimately leading you to have papules and pustules. In even more severe cases, the follicle walls may burst in the later stages of this inflammation. Lipids, fatty acids, corneocytes, bacteria, and cell fragments being released and causing even more inflammation to the surrounding skin.

So, with all this, it is always good to keep in mind that the oiliness of your skin and possible acne flare-ups that you may find yourself overwhelmed by, may have nothing to do with the fact that your skin is merely oily. Consider also that the oiliness of your skin may change depending on the time of year and minor changes in weather.

If you find that you are battling any of these things daily since you have discovered you have oily skin, here are a few things that you can do to make it a little more bearable for you.
- Wash your skin, especially the skin on your face, no more than twice a day and only extra after you have sweat quite a bit.
- Use a gentle cleanser and do not scrub.
- Please refrain from picking, popping, or squeezing your pimples. I don't care if you have just washed your hands. The makeup of the bacteria on your fingers is different from the PH of the bacteria on your face. Ultimately causing an alteration in the composition of the sebum on your face, creating not only more breakouts, but causing the papules or pustules to take longer to heal.
- Also, look for the word "noncomedogenic" on your skincare and make-up products. It means that these products are not intended to clog your pores. They are also considered to be

less toxic. So, if you are suffering from inflammation, the last thing you need is to expose your face to more toxins.

COMBINATION SKIN

Now that we have discussed three of the most common skin types, it is now time to review, probably one of the more common of the three but less talked about skin types — Combination Skin.

First of all, what is a Combination Skin? Simply put, combination skin types usually vary in the T-zone (forehead, nose, and chin) and cheek areas of a person's face. A person's T-zone can differ substantially from a very slim zone to a very extended area. Many people often misidentify combination skin with oily skin, because it is frequently characterized by a greasy T-zone area, enlarged or inflamed pores that sport some impurities, but normal to dry cheeks. It is only by this that combination skin is usually determined, (i.e. by the T-zone being slightly or more than somewhat oilier than the rest of the face). Also, the cheeks are often dryer.

The leading causes and contributors to combination skin are not as many or extensive as the other three, and this is why it's less discussed than others. But just because there isn't that much material to be said for combination skin as opposed to its counterparts, it does not necessarily make it any less critical. Just seemingly less prevalent than others because its explanation seems to be simpler than the rest. The oilier parts of combination skin are caused by an overproduction of sebum, as you probably guessed from what you read earlier. While the drier areas of the face are caused by a lack thereof, ultimately correlating to a lipid deficiency.

SKIN HEALTH

The overall health of a person's skin can change drastically over the course of their life because there are many different internal as well as external factors at play that determine the condition of someone's skin; factors such as, climate and pollution, medication, stress, hereditary considerations that influence levels of sebum production or lack thereof, sweat, other natural moisturizing factors that your skin produces. Not to mention, the products you use daily and the skincare choices that you make, or don't. All of these play a huge part in the overall health and good or bad condition of your skin.

Skincare products should always be chosen to match an individual's unique skin type as it applies to them, as well as addressing the condition of their skin. Dermatologists and other skincare experts and professionals such as myself, determine a person's skin type and condition by measuring the following factors. First and foremost, signs of aging. As we all know, our skin type can evolve over the course of our lifetime, due to things like age. For example, a person with an oily skin type in their adolescent years can often find that their skin is becoming much drier after puberty. Similarly, those blessed with well-balanced skin can also discover that their skin is becoming rapidly drier or possibly exhibiting more signs of inflammation as they age.

As all skin types are not impervious to the grasp of time and age, skin tends to lose its volume and density over time; revealing things such as fine lines and wrinkles, or changes in pigmentation and color. So, it is the understanding and measurement of these signs that help us to determine the condition of our skin.

SKIN COLOR

Skin color and ethnicity is something that influences how our skin health. It reacts to different external forces in nature, such as the sun, pigmentation disorders, various irritations, and inflammations. A person's primary skin color is determined by the density of the epidermis and the distribution of melanin throughout an individual's skin.

The redness of a person's skin is also a useful measure of skin condition. It indicates how adequate your circulation is, and this is quite helpful in identifying skin conditions such as couperose and rosacea.

SEBUM AND SWEAT PRODUCTION

The level of sebum that is produced by the sebaceous glands in your skin controls the effectiveness of your skin's defensive mechanisms, and as a consequence, the condition of your skin. As you previously learned, the overproduction of sebum can lead to oily skin that is at risk for acne and other blemishes; while low sebum contributes to drier skin. The perspiratory glands in your skin produce sweat to assist the body in keeping its optimum temperature. Much like how air conditioning in your car or home influences the overall temperature and how you function in either place, excessive or low sweat production significantly affects the condition and functionality of your skin.

NMF's

Natural moisturizing factors, or NMF's such as amino acids, are naturally produced in healthy, well-balanced skin. They assist the skin in the retention of the amount of water it needs, and also contribute to the maintenance of its elasticity and suppleness. When the skin's protective barrier is compromised, it is often unable to hold on to these essentials. Thus, causing the skin's moisture to decrease and ultimately affecting the condition of the skin itself.

With all of these factors at play, determining just what skin type you have and its condition on your own can tend to be a bit overwhelming at times. You may find that you display several, if not all, of these different traits when it comes to your skin at different times, causing you to be even more confused about the best approach to determining precisely what skin type you have.

In pursuit of that healthy glow, you'd also want to know what issues your skin is currently enduring, and how best to manage all of those things in the interest of your skin's overall health. Again, my advice to you is that the first step you need to take is to find a reputable dermatologist as well as an aesthetician, and allow them to help you to safely and accurately determine, not only, your skin type; but the overall condition of your skin. We are works of art, and as we all know; no two pieces of craftsmanship are precisely alike. We are all one of a kind. Therefore, our individual deserves and needs unique individual care. So do what is best for your skin by finding out what unique story it has to tell you about keeping it healthy.

CHAPTER 3

SENSITIVE SKIN AND HOW TO TREAT IT

Blotchy redness, the appearance of a rash, overall dryness of small or large areas, stinging, itching and burning sensations. All of the above point towards a skin more conditioned to sensitivity. There is a bit of an argument over whether this should be considered a skin type in itself, rather than just classifying it as a skin condition. However, there are many contributing factors causing skin sensitivity in pretty much anyone without a well-balanced canvas of skin.

It is more logical to take it for what it is, and what this is ultimately, is a skin condition. To buttress, it is something that can be managed over time and eventually cured, as opposed to a person's skin type which is always evolving and changing. Plus, you cannot necessarily cure someone of having a particular skin type. It is something they are genetically inclined to have, meaning they are born with it, rather than something that flares up from time to time.

There is no particular definition for sensitive skin. It occurs when the skin's natural barrier is altered, causing water loss and allowing for the penetration of compromising irritants. The majority of people in the medical community believe it to be skin that is irritated by things that don't bother most people. This category of most people being people who have well-balanced skin. However, determining whether you fall into the classification of the population of humanity that has sensitive skin is quite simple. If your skin burns, itches, or gets red and inflamed after you apply particular make-up or skincare products; these are all excellent signs that you have sensitive skin. The more complicated part, however, is figuring just what is causing this sensitivity. Some people, find these signs are symptoms of an allergy or a mild form of a skin disorder like that of eczema or rosacea. Its symptoms often become exacerbated by most things we expose our skin to daily — everything from the sun to some ingredients in cosmetics and cleansers. However, it is often in response to particular chemicals found in unnatural skincare products.

Drugstores, supermarkets, salons, and spa shelves have no shortage of make-up, cleansers, and lotions that are labeled explicitly for people with sensitive skin. However, how can you be sure if you can or should use these products on yourself? Also, if you do indeed really have sensitive skin, will they help you? If you find that your skin is sensitive, try to determine what the triggers are for your particular skin so that you can avoid them in the future. Also, your doctor, as well as your dermatologist, should be able to assist you, if you are currently having these questions and issues, or if you discover that a specific skincare product is a cause.

For many people in the world's population, sensitive skin can seem like a permanent condition; unlike others who find that certain internal or external factors only trigger their sensitivity. So, there is not a definite or particular skin-care rule to follow for everyone when it comes to this subject. However, some products can cause more havoc than others. So, here are some basic guidelines to help make living with your sensitive skin, a little bit easier and more manageable.

First of all, avoid fragrances, especially anything that is heavily fragranced. Scented soap, lotion, and liquid cleansers more times than not have ingredients that cause irritation and inflammation of the skin. Cosmetic companies and the like aren't required by law to list chemicals on labels of their products, or general ingredients at all; which go into making their fragrances. It makes it much harder to pinpoint and keep track of exactly which ones are the cause of your irritation.

What about scented products with so-called all-natural ingredients, like essential oils or plant-based botanicals? You ask. Just because something is labeled "natural", does not mean that your skin will not react to it. If something has been labeled USDA organic, it must only contain materials that were grown organically from the ground. You honestly do not need fragrance from your lotion or soaps, so for those of you with sensitive skin, it maybe is best to avoid scented things all together until you can discover the real culprit of your issue.

However, we are not exactly out of the woods yet. Even products labeled as unscented are crafted with chemicals, to mask the smell of their active ingredients with firm odor profiles. So instead of merely looking for products that say unscented, instead look for products that are labeled "fragrance free", which means that they have no scent whatsoever, not even a masking ingredient. This rule applies to all soaps and lotions, along with other products that may come into contact with your skin during your day to day life — things like shampoos, household cleaners, deodorant, and especially laundry detergent.

Be sure to watch out for those pesky preservatives. Chemicals called parabens are added to things like lotions and other cosmetics to prevent the growth of bacteria from making them last longer. The reason for this is not to benefit you. They do this so that they do not have to spend quite so much money making more of the product, because it can last longer on the shelves while waiting to be purchased. It is why I made such a big deal about checking expiration dates on your products because they do matter. You are putting this stuff on your body; most importantly, it is going on your face. These preservative ingredients may cause issues with people who have sensitive skin. If you find that you have had an adverse reaction to products containing ingredients like propylparaben or butylparaben, try switching to specifically paraben-free products. Other components to watch out for include methylchloroisothiazolinone and methylisothiazolinone. These preservatives are the most common causes of skin irritation and allergies in their users.

Another suggestion would be to skip the toner. I like to tell my clients who have skin that is easily irritated, to avoid all alcohol-based toners and astringents of any kind. These are designed to remove oil and dirt. However, seeing as how there is much overlap between dry skin and sensitive skin, and that the former usually in most cases tends to lead to the latter, products with alcohol in them can be very destructive for both. Toners are not a necessary part of most people's skincare routine, just as long as you are making sure to wash your face at least once to twice a day with a liquid cleanser that is appropriate for you. For people with sensitive or dry skin, I recommend skipping the toner entirely. If you find yourself a bit wary about this suggestion, I recommend also speaking with a dermatologist or aesthetician about suggesting something that would be a gentler alternative.

Find what works for you and what does not. Everyone's sensitivities are as unique as their skin, and no two are alike. So feel free to try one new product at a time, until you figure out what works for you and what does not. Just because your sister or your mom may have sensitive skin and they can or cannot use a particular product, the same rule may not apply to your skin. Also, remember while making changes to help manage your sensitive skin, take it slowly. Many people often, when they discover that they do have a sensitivity to one product, will renovate their entire skincare routine all at once. There may be one specific product or ingredient to blame for their discomfort or pain, or a mixture of these things that do not work well together. However, they will not be able to figure this out because they decided to go ahead and throw everything away and get new stuff. Newer stuff may contain the same or different ingredients that can cause another adverse reaction altogether. So I suggest introducing one new product at a time. Try it out, wait a few weeks, and see if it helps or makes the problem worse. If your dermatologist or aesthetician recommends something new, be sure to make them aware of the products that you already use regularly, and what your reactions to those things are, whether they are good or bad.

I am in no way saying at all that people with sensitive skin should avoid wearing make-up. Even if you have had some adverse reactions in the past to different cosmetics, this means that you need to find the right products that work best with your skin, which granted, can take some trial and error. So, choose your make-up carefully. Avoid products with fragrances and preservatives, and look for make-up that is formulated with ingredients that are oil-free and non-comedogenic. As I have said before, this means that the product is designed to not clog your pores, which can lead to other such inflammatory disorders such as acne, while causing flare-ups of skin sensitivity. Also, be sure to wash your face before you go to bed. Sleeping in your make-up can cause even worse irritation and breakouts.

It is also vital for those of you with sensitive skin to protect yourselves from the sun. However, sunblock tends to be able to irritate your sensitive just as well, if not worse than the sun itself. So, what do you do? I would highly recommend using a physical sunblock. There are two most common types of sunscreen on the market at the moment, chemical and physical. The first type is made up of chemicals like oxybenzone, avobenzone, and octocrylene; which are meant to absorb the sun's rays and break them down. The second type is what we call physical because it uses more tiny mineral compounds, such as zinc and titanium. These things sit on top of your skin and deflect the sun's rays. Many people are quite capable of using either of these types of sunblock with absolutely no problems at all. However, then again, some have allergic reactions in the form of skin sensitivity to these chemical blockers. The ultraviolet radiation can combine with chemicals in the sunscreen or sunblock, and trigger a rash or a blister when a person goes out into the sun.

So for this reason, I highly recommend that if you fall into the category of someone who has sensitive skin, choose a physical sunscreen or sunblock with only the active ingredients of zinc oxide or titanium oxide, as these will be better safe than sorry. Also remember to avoid sunscreens that have fragrances, oils, and any para-aminobenzoic acid (PABA), which is another common allergen and irritant.

Your dermatologist will often be able to assist you in deciphering if any new development you have is a treatable condition, or just only sensitivity to something in your skincare regiment. Even if you have not switched to new products lately, one of them could very well still be the culprit. This is true because your body must be exposed to something for some time, before it becomes aware that there is an allergy developing. Just as our taste buds change entirely every seven years, so do our cells. Also, another thing to keep in mind is that manufacturers can, and often do frequently, change the ingredients in the formula of a product without making the consumer aware of it. So, for your safety and comfort, be sure to be always aware of labels and expiration dates on your skincare and cosmetic products.

CHAPTER 4

WHY REGULAR FACIALS AND A PERSONAL AESTHETICIAN ARE AS IMPORTANT AS GOING TO THE DENTIST

Somehow over the centuries people have unfortunately gotten the idea put into their heads that facials are only something that you should do when you are looking to treat yourself. A luxury, one whose benefits are saved for only those who are rich and famous enough to afford or need such things, to keep them looking young and beautiful in the public eye. And, yeah let's get real, they do tend to be a bit pricey. But then again, so is a trip to the doctor or the dentist. You consider these things to be priorities as opposed to luxuries that you just allow yourself every once in a while, when you want to feel bougie or pampered, right? Also, take a moment to think about where your money is really spent instead. Is getting a regular that much more expensive in the long run? Perhaps, I would even go as far as to say, it is worth more of your time than whatever it is you are replacing it with instead. You get your teeth cleaned and serviced, you try to remember to floss, and believe that it is important to go to the dentist for a routine clean; you go to the doctor for a physical, and they recommend that you drink plenty of liquids, get 6-8 hours of sleep, and remember to exercise, and you oblige. So why not go to an aesthetician and get a regular facial? When your skin is one of the most important organs of your body, aside from your heart, brain, and lungs. It is the guardian and first defense against outside free radicals, pollutants, and contagions. Why don't we see how important it is to take care of it, and treat it with the respect it deserves? It has been there for you since the time you were born, and now it is time that you be there for it.

Until I got into this career, I did not truly understand just how extraordinary of an amount of toxins, dirt, grease, grime, and dead skin cells accumulate on the human face. Unfortunately, unless you live in a bubble, this kind of build is an inevitable and unavoidable occurrence of everyday living. Granted, there are many things that we do to keep our skin clean. However, this is not always enough. This is why I and so many others compare and vehemently advocate, that getting a facial is of the same crucial importance as going to the dentist or the doctor. We have to make it a point to get a routine annual physical, to keep track of how our health is doing as we age. Keeping up with such appointments, many would agree, saves us a lot of money in the long term when it comes to our teeth or the rest of our physical body. Consider how much more something like a root canal or an abscess extraction costs in comparison to a routine clean and maintenance check.

Your skin, like your teeth, needs to be cleaned and evaluated regularly by someone who is a properly trained professional, to maintain not only a healthy complexion, but preserve the overall health of the rest of your skin. An aesthetician should be viewed as the dentist or doctor for your skin. Once you have realized this to be the truth, you will see how getting a facial on a frequent basis, even if it is just once every few months, or say two to three times a year; will save you from needless spending on your skin in the future.

Some of the biggest benefits of getting a regular facial, you will notice, are that your make-up will go on more smoothly and evenly. In fact, you may even find yourself surprised by just how little an amount of make-up you need to apply to your face, the more you keep in the routine of getting a facial. A facial will also help you to make sure that you are getting the most for your money, as far as skin care products and your at-home skin routine are concerned. Your aesthetician will deeply clean and exfoliate your face. This will allow all of the products used to fully absorb into your skin for optimal, beneficial results; thus creating a good, clean slate foundation of skin for you to continue your at-home skin care maintenance routine with.

When it comes to guarding against the signs of premature aging, or just signs of aging in general, facials are one of the best possible treatments you can receive. Treating yourself to a facial on a regular basis will decrease your risk of having to shell out the big bucks for high dollar procedures and injections, that will not have lasting effects. At least not beneficial lasting effects. I think you all know to what I am referring. You will find that a facial will improve the skin's overall tone, texture, elasticity, and suppleness by acting as an antidote against the damaging effects of prolonged sun exposure and air pollution.

Exfoliation is one of the most important steps of a facial. When you have a professional exfoliate the skin on your face, this usually includes some form of microdermabrasion or having some kind of fruit acid peel to assist in removing the dead skin cells from your face. This part of the process acts as a kickstart for the cell turnover process, encouraging the new growth and cultivation of new more vibrant cells, and allowing healthier, more alive cells to take the place of those that are being shed away by the process. Receiving a regular exfoliation from a professional often works wonders on those who are looking to diminish the appearance of acne scarring and even signs of aging. Not only is this part of the process highly beneficial, there is also a facial massage that is included with every facial. The massage itself works miracles on wrinkled, tired, or scarred skin. Not many people believe that there is an actual science to the way a face needs to be massaged in order for it to be most beneficial. In fact, if a massage is done incorrectly, especially a facial massage, it can do far more harm than good. It can not only lead to sagging or stretched skin, but encourage the flood of toxins back into your face rather than out. Because, one of the facts about a facial massage is that when done correctly, it encourages the drainage of the lymphatic glands, flushing out the toxins, and all the while promoting healthy blood and fluid circulation.

Last but most certainly not least, the absolutely best part of getting a facial is that the results are practically instant. You will find yourself hard pressed to come across the path of a skin treatment or skin care or cosmetic product that will live up to society's high expectations. However, after only one facial, there will be evidence of an immediate improvement in the appearance of your skin.

These are just a few of the reasons that I find to be highly important, with regards to making regular facials a priority.

CHAPTER 5

BAD SKIN CARE HABITS VS HEALTHY SKIN CARE HABITS

Your make-up will only look as good as the skin that it is dressing. I know that I have voiced this particular sentiment before, and many of you listened. And, you are reading this book because you desire to treat your skin right, so that it looks as good as it possibly can. But there are some daily routines that a lot of you still have when it comes to how you treat your skin, that you may not think about, in terms of how they add up to sometimes irreversible skin damage over time. So, I am writing this chapter to help you keep track of how you are treating your complexion, so that you will know what habits to keep and which ones to change.

First, you have that pesky habit of not washing your face before bed. I understand the urge to skip the sink, probably more than anyone, after a long day at work. But just because you do not see the dirt and the grime on your face does not mean that it is not there. And, over time your complexion will most certainly pay the price for it. Oil, dirt, and free flying toxins build up over time, and lead to both inflammations and ultimately breakouts. So my friends, wash your face and say your prayers, because germs and Jesus are everywhere!

Use a gentle cleanser with moisturizers such as glycerin or botanical oils to keep your complexion hydrated. But if there just so happens to be a time where you find that you cannot get to a sink before heading off to bed, a few swipes with a facial cleansing wipe will do the trick.

Second, if you smoke, you should know that nicotine and carbon dioxide reduce blood flow to your skin. Which means it does not get enough oxygen or nutrients. Also, the chemicals in tobacco damage the collagen elastin proteins that give your skin its structure. A person who smokes for prolonged periods of time tends to have thinner, duller, skin that is more wrinkled, and slower to heal than those who do not smoke. Not to mention, the years of puckering your lips to hold a cigarette or squinting your eyes to keep out the smoke, may deepen the already appearing lines and lead to even more and deeper wrinkles in those areas and others. While some antioxidants that can be found in things like vitamins A and C can ease some of the damage; the only fool proof way to fix the damage before it is too late is to quit for good as soon as you can.

Thirdly, you either skimp on the sunscreen or sunblock, or just completely ignore it altogether. Sunshine may feel very good on your skin, and it is very beneficial in moderate doses. Especially as it helps your body to properly assimilate vitamins such as C, D, E, B, and A, but sometimes, there can be too much of a good thing. Because for all of its benefits, it also possesses UV rays that can over time of prolonged exposure, lead to things such as premature aging and some types of skin cancer. And, it is not only on beach days when you need the most protection. The sun can damage your skin even when it is cold or cloudy outside. Using a broad-spectrum SPF blocks both UVA and UVB rays, and keeps you fully protected. So look for a minimum of SPF 30, and when you are outside for long periods of time, plan to reapply at least every 2 hours as recommended. Be sure that you are using enough. A full-size teaspoon is just about the right amount for your entire face including your hairline, around your nose, and down under your chin.

Next, you eat a lot of processed sugars, trans fats, and empty carbs. Not enough fruits, vegetables, or lean meats. Many studies have shown the correlation between diets that are heavy in sugar and their ability to speed up the aging process, due to the unsurmountable amount of stress that these diets place on the human body. They cause the body to become insulin resistant, storing fat everywhere that it can, particularly your internal organs, and creating a whole other host of problems that reach far beyond just a problem with acne or premature aging. Many people with these kinds of diets have succumbed to various life-threatening ailments and diseases, simply because their diet was not what it should have been to properly care for their body. What I mean by processed sugars is simple, I am talking about sweet treats like candy, ice cream, as well as starches in refined carbs that turn straight into sugar as soon as they make it to your blood stream. Things like white bread and pasta, or white potatoes. A more skin friendly diet, as well as body friendly diet, should focus on things like vegetables, fruits, whole grains, and lots of lean meat. As well as a healthy amount of some animal fats, as these are needed for good cognitive function as well as cell regeneration. They actually give you the ability to age gracefully, and people begin to wonder how you've come to look so much younger than you are. Produce, especially fresh produce, also provides antioxidants that can help to repair your skin. So eat better for your skin's sake, if not just your waistline.

Next up, I know, I know, you have a pimple the size of a small volcano brewing on your face, and you want it to go away right this second. However, popping this sucker is not the answer. Popping your pimples leads to scarring and more infection, which leads to more pimples. What about a cream instead? I find in situations like this that there are two very helpful agents that have proven themselves to be quite effective. Benzoyl peroxide and salicylic acid are two of the most effective things that you can use in this instance. But do keep in mind that different products have differing levels of these ingredients. And, many people would be tempted to reach for the highest dosage right away, thinking that it will be the most beneficial when it comes to getting rid of their pesky blight right this minute. I am here to tell you that despite however much you may be tempted; you may not need to cave. Various studies have proven that only 2.5% benzoyl peroxide is just as effective if not more than 5% or 10%. So the term less is more really does apply here. Plus, higher concentrations of such medications can lead to even more irritation and inflammation, particularly if your skin is already sensitive. This could lead your complexion to take on an even angrier look than before you did this. So, nothing more than a 2.5% benzoyl peroxide, and as for the salicylic acid 2% is gentle but effective enough for most people. However, if you do find yourself flaring up even at these levels of concentration; try lowering the concentration just a bit more, and it might help.

One of my biggest, if not the biggest pet peeve I have, is people exfoliating their flakey skin themselves. Scales and flakes are the first signs of dryness. Even though exfoliating will slough away any loose patches of dead skin that you have in that particular spot, the rough treatment of this part of your skin can actually create a disruption in the barrier that balances the moisture level in your skin. So instead of scrubbing this away vigorously, soothe the dryness rather with some form of hydration. A preferably fragrance-free lotion or cream with a moisturizer like glycerin, petrolatum, and butter like cocoa or shea which absorb into the skin quickly, and leave the skin quenched without leaving it greasy.

All is not lost though, there are some other habits with which you can change these unruly things out. Better habits to lead you onto the path of treating your skin better so that it will look as good as you dream it will. An important thing to keep in mind is that your skin reflects your overall health on the outside. So in order to take care of your skin, you must build up healthy habits for the rest of your body, too.

First, stay clean! Remember to wash your face at least twice a day, once in the morning and once at night before bed. After you cleanse your skin, follow up with a toner and moisturizer. Toners help to remove fine traces of oil, dirt, and makeup you may have missed when cleansing. Look for a moisturizer geared toward your skin type; dry, normal, or oily. Yes, even oily skin can benefit from a moisturizer. You would be surprised.

As I mentioned earlier in this chapter, over exposure to the UV radiation from the sun can cause many changes in your skin's condition. Age spots, benign growths, some not so benign growths such as carcinomas and melanoma, color changes, freckles, and wrinkles. It is important to note here that the majority of skin cancers come from prolonged sun exposure. So make sure that you are wisely limiting your time outside, especially during the brightest part of the day which is between 10am and 2pm. Always wear a broad-spectrum sunscreen with the physical blocker zinc oxide and a sun protection factor (SPF) of 30 or greater. Wear protective clothing, like a long-sleeved shirt, pants, and a wide-brimmed hat.

Also, last but not least, remember to check yourself. Pay attention to your skin and the messages your body is trying to send you through it. Be vigilant so that you will notice if there are any sudden or adverse changes to any moles or patches on your skin that could indicate any type of skin cancer. And, feel free to use the tools at your disposal, such as a dermatologist or primary physician if you have any questions as to whether you should be concerned about the sudden changes; should you happen to find any.

CHAPTER 6

HOW TO BUILD YOUR OWN AT HOME SKIN CARE ROUTINE

The most important step to begin with in building your at-home skin care routine is first establishing what type of skin you have.

STEP 1: KNOW YOUR SKIN TYPE

The right routine starts with knowing what kind of skin you have. Then you'll know how to take care of it.
* Dry skin is flaky, scaly, or rough.
* Oily skin is shiny, greasy, and may have big pores.
* Combination skin is dry in some spots (cheeks) and oily in others (forehead, nose, and chin).
- Normal skin is balanced, clear, and not sensitive.

I know that sensitive skin is not a type necessarily, but for this instance we will put it in step one so that it will be something you keep in mind while determining your skin's condition.

STEP 2: CLEANING YOUR SKIN PROPERLY

When Should You Wash?

You can dry your skin by washing it too much, so once a day is fine for most people. In the morning, rinse your face with lukewarm water. Use a soft towel to pat it dry. At night, wash with a cleanser or gentle soap to get rid of the day's dirt and makeup. If you exercise, play sports, or have PE, you may want to wash your face afterward with a gentle cleanser. Sweat can clog your pores and cause acne or make it worse.

NORMAL/COMBO SKIN

Don't just grab whatever soap is in the shower or at the sink to wash your face. And don't feel like you have to buy fancy, expensive products, either. Just find skin care that works for you. Apply a gentle cleanser or soap with your fingertips. Don't scrub your face. Rinse with plenty of warm water, then pat dry. If your skin dries out or gets oily, try a different cleanser.

CLEANING DRY SKIN

For this skin type, use a gentle cleanser that doesn't have alcohol or fragrances. Those ingredients can dry you out even more. Gently wash your skin, then rinse with plenty of warm water. Don't use hot water -- it removes the natural oils from your face faster. Try exfoliating once a week to get rid of flaky skin cells. It will make your skin look clearer and more even.

CLEANING OILY SKIN

Use an oil-free foaming cleanser to wash your face. Rinse with plenty of warm water. You may want to use a toner or astringent after, but be careful because it might irritate your skin. These products can remove extra oil, which makes your face less shiny, and help keep skin clean.

CLEANING SENSITIVE SKIN

Wash your face with a gentle cleanser and rinse with warm water. Don't rub your skin with a towel -- gently pat it dry. Exfoliating may irritate sensitive skin. Try not to use products that have alcohol, soap, acid, or fragrance. Instead, look on the label for calming ingredients like aloe, chamomile, green tea polyphenols, and oats. The fewer ingredients in a product, the happier your face will be.

HOW TO TREAT ACNE

Don't pop those pimples! That can lead to infection and scars. Instead, try acne-fighting products. They come as lotions, creams, gels, and cleansing pads. Follow the directions carefully. If you use them too much or too often, they can irritate your skin and cause more blemishes. Keep in mind you will need to be patient, some of these products can take 8 weeks to work. If your acne is really bad, seek help from a dermatologist.
However, while you're waiting, you may still be looking for a way to make them disappear, even if it's just temporarily through the magic of make-up. In order to make zits less noticeable, you can

cover them with oil-free makeup. Foundation may help cover large patches of acne. Concealer covers smaller areas. Green-tinted color-correcting concealer may cancel out redness. You also can hide acne and treat it at the same time. Some tinted creams and concealers contain salicylic acid or benzoyl peroxide. Stop using any product, if it bothers your skin or causes more acne.

STEP 3: MOISTURIZE

You may think you're too young to need moisturizer, or your skin is too oily; but all skin types need one every day. Apply it while your skin is still damp from washing or rinsing, to help seal in the moisture. If you have acne or your skin is oily, find a moisturizer that's lightweight and oil-free, so it won't block your pores.

STEP 4: SUNSCREEN

Your moisturizer may already have sunscreen in it. But it's a good idea to use separate protection, too. The sun can damage your skin in only 15 minutes. Look for a sunscreen that gives broad-spectrum protection with an SPF of at least 30. Wear it every day, even if it's not sunny and even if it's cold. Reapply every 2 hours.

Bonus Tips:

DANGERS OF TANNING

You may like to tan, but you hurt your skin when it changes color from too much exposure to the sun or indoor tanning. Prolonged UV exposure can make you more likely to get skin cancer, now or later. It can also lead to wrinkly, leathery-looking skin and spots. Regularly using tanning beds raises your chances of getting melanoma, the deadliest skin cancer, by 8 times.

FAKE TANS

For a safer tanning experience, try sunless self-tanner. It stains your skin and comes in many forms, including lotions, sprays, and towelettes. Or try airbrush tanning, where a salon expert sprays the tan right on your skin. For a quick fake tan, try some bronzer. It's a brush-on powder or tinted cream that gives the look of a fresh tan. But remember, you'll still need to protect your skin from the sun.

These are just a few of the building blocks to setting up a healthier and more conscientious at home skin care routine between regular visits to your aesthetician.

CHAPTER 7

ALL-NATURAL SKIN CARE INGREDIENTS

Just because the world today now seems to be brimming with high tech devices and so-called cutting-edge ingredients, does not mean that when it comes to handling some of the most prevalent skin care issues that newer is necessarily better. In many cases, you will find that simple, more natural options, are far more effective than scientifically engineered solutions made to support big Pharma.

Here are some of the ingredients that I have found to really be the best of both worlds as far as skin care is concerned. Both naturally based and scientifically supported.

COCONUT OIL

Benefits: Hydration, anti-inflammatory.

There's a growing science supporting the use of this plant fat as a topical skin soother. Recent research has shown that coconut oil can suppress some of the body's natural inflammatory agents, while making the skin a better barrier. Many people love using coconut oil products to help fight dry, itchy skin and skin diseases such as eczema and psoriasis. Some psoriasis patients swear by overnight coconut oil scalp treatments worn under a plastic shower cap. I would just be careful about using copious amounts of coconut oil in blemish or acne prone areas of your skin as the oil may prove to be too dense and clog the pores in those areas.

GOTU KOLA (CENTELLA ASIATICA)

Benefits: Wound healing.

This ancient herb, often used in Asian cuisine, is now a part of modern skin care due to its wound-healing benefits. Chemicals in the plant boost blood supply to injury sites and strengthen the skin. Researchers have found that when skin injuries in rats are treated with Centella asiatica, the sites showed higher rates of healing. The combination of amino acids, beta carotene, fatty acids, and phytochemicals helped to speed healing time exponentially, making it a more helpful way to treat injuries.

GREEN TEA

Benefits: Sun protection, anti-aging.

The connection between drinking green tea and improved health has been suggested for centuries, and many people swear by this. But it may also help to use the plant on the skin. Green tea has been found to have good results in terms of photoprotection and anti-aging benefits. The polyphenols in green tea have antioxidant properties as well as soothing abilities that help treat sun-damaged skin and offer a way to address the signs of sun damage.

OATMEAL

Benefits: Anti-inflammatory, eczema relief.

Oatmeal contains anti-inflammatory and anti-irritant chemicals called avenanthramides. It also has moisturizing beta glucans and starches. It's the reason why oatmeal baths are so effective for conditions like eczema and rashes. But not all oatmeal is created equal.

Colloidal oatmeal is a powder that's derived from grinding and preparing oats into very tiny particles. This size and quality of oats is what makes the ingredient so therapeutic, and able to blend with water to form the soothing paste when mixed together.

I like colloidal oatmeal products because they're gentle and safe, and studies show they don't tend to cause allergies or undue irritation in people with sensitive skin issues. Many dermatologists have discovered that if their eczema patients develop gentle skin care habits and regularly slather on a thick moisturizer containing colloidal oatmeal, they don't need topical steroids as much or as often. And sometimes, they're even able to completely forego the use of medications when it comes to treating their skin issues altogether.

SHEA BUTTER

Benefits: Anti-inflammatory, itch relief.

Derived from the nut of a shea tree, shea butter is an active ingredient in many moisturizers. It hydrates skin effectively because it is loaded with fatty acids. These nutrients have a calming and anti-inflammatory effect on the skin. Shea butter might be most useful for treating and soothing eczema. Clinical studies using shea butter as a treatment for eczema in children showed less itching within as soon as 4 weeks, and another study with adults showed improvement in as little as 2 weeks. Another plus of this natural moisturizer I would like to point out is this: Shea butter doesn't seem to cause skin allergies, which makes it right even for the most sensitive skin types.

SOY

Benefits: Inhibits pigmentation, improves collagen production.

Soybeans contain a variety of plant-based chemicals that impact the skin. Among them are antioxidants, fatty acids, and isoflavones. The legume also produces estrogens or phytoestrogens that address skin conditions related to menopause. One of the reasons it is believed that a woman's skin brightness decreases after menopause, is because of decreased estrogen. Some topical estrogens have been shown to help decrease UV-induced pigmentation and can improve collagen synthesis. Even though soy does not offer as robust of a result as retinoids, it is still another option for women who are looking to address these conditions. The isoflavones in soy also offer sun protection that can help address pigmentation to keep skin even.

TEA TREE OIL

Benefits: Anti-microbial, blemish-fighting.

The herbal remedy derived from tea tree leaves has antimicrobial and anti-inflammatory effects that help combat a range of germs, fungus, and bacteria. Because of these properties, tea tree oil helps combat bacteria driven acne; which means it will greatly help reduce inflammatory types of blemishes, pustules, and other inflamed papules. Even though topical treatment in moderate amounts has proven to be quite effective.

It is important to keep in mind that tea tree oil is very potent and can cause some irritation and redness if over used. So be sure to dilute the tea tree oil with something before using directly on skin. Also, make sure that you are monitoring areas of your skin for signs of redness or burning after using this oil, due to the fact that you may be over using it in these particular areas and need to take a break for a little while.

Just some final thoughts before closing this chapter and moving onto the fun part, where I teach you how to put everything that you have learned into effective action at home for yourself. I would just like to say that as with any sort of new endeavor that involves bettering your health; like with starting a new diet or exercise regime, skin care in many ways is the same, and it is always a good idea to run these ideas by your dermatologist and aesthetician first before going forward with something like this. Not so they can talk you out of it by any means, I am just saying that it is most likely that not only will they encourage you to take these steps; but they will also be there to answer any questions that you have and give you helpful warnings and instructions as you need them.

CHAPTER 8

MAKING YOUR OWN SKIN CARE PRODUCTS

One of the best ways to take control of your skin care regimen and know exactly what goes into your skin care products, is to *make them yourself*. This way you can be more confident about your personal safety and overall health of your skin, because you crafted these tools yourself. This principle covers many things and not just skin care. But for now, that is what we will focus on.

Making your own skin care products means you can forget about worrying about the cost of expensive, and possibly harmful, department store facial cleansers and other such products. For instance, the first recipe I will be teaching you is a face wash; one that you can easily make for only two dollars, with ingredients that you most likely already have in your pantry. Not to mention, it is a far more nourishing and beneficial face wash than you will find in any department store, and it is guaranteed to be safe for all skin types. Even for those with particular skin sensitivities.

I know it may be pretty embarrassing to admit at first, how we all used to think before now that a high-quality facial cleanser or any other such product meant that it had to cost quite a pretty penny. I know of many people who are still shelling out upwards of thirty dollars for department store brand skin care products. These products are in containers that only yield anywhere from 2-6 ounces worth of product a pop. Only lasting the person maybe a month or so, if they were lucky. But this is not the only ridiculous thing, many people shell out even more than that if they are looking to purchase an entire skin care regimen of cleanser, toner, and moisturizer, thinking that somehow their skin would benefit from these products simply because they were so expensive. They go by the old adage of, "you get what you pay for". Even though this is certainly a true philosophy to go by, it does not necessarily mean that the payment itself has to be monetary. You can get just as good of a quality of product, if not better, from something that you have invested your mental and physical time and energy in. You can also rest assured that the end products will be made without any harsh chemicals or preservatives, often found in name brands that fall short on their promise to not be harmful you. This is why the tools that you create yourself are far more effective than those that you simply buy from a store. You are putting your energy into it, all the while hopefully listening to what your body is telling you instinctually that it needs.

That being said, here are just a few ways to get started with making your own skin care and beauty products, like face wash, cleanser, toner, and moisturizers.

FACE WASH

You just need liquid castile soap, water, essential oils and carrier oil.

Ingredients

- 3/4 cup cooled organic brewed chamomile tea (or filtered or distilled water)
- 1/4 cup liquid castile soap
- 1/2 tsp organic almond oil
- 3-4 drops vitamin E oil optional
- 8 drops Frankincense essential oil
- 8 drops Lavender essential oil

Instructions

1. In a 4 to 6 oz. foaming soap bottle, add liquid Castile soap, organic almond oil and vitamin E oil.
2. Add essential oils as needed.
3. Fill with chamomile tea or water to the top of the bottle.
4. Shake well and use as needed.

HOW TO USE THIS FACIAL CLEANSER

1. Shake bottle well.
2. Wet face with warm water.
3. Add 2-3 pumps of DIY Face Wash to the palm of your hand and then use both hands to massage onto the face.
4. Massage face for about 1 minute.
5. Rinse with warm water.
6. Follow with this DIY Facial Serum.

FACE SCRUB

The great thing about this recipe is the fact that it is so simple. It is pretty much just putting essential oils into baking soda, and then storing it in an airtight container of some sort. My favorite essential oils for this particular recipe are Frankincense and Lavender, because both are very gentle on the skin, as well as great for helping with your skin's overall tone and texture.

Ingredients

1. 1/2 cup baking soda
2. 8 drops of Frankincense
3. 8 drops of Lavender
4. Water

Instructions

Mix all ingredients and store in a small jar.

HOW TO USE

1. Use 1-2 teaspoons at a time and add water to make a paste.
2. Lightly massage the paste onto your skin to gently exfoliate the face for a couple of minutes.
3. Rinse off.

FACE MASKS

With these at home organic face masks you can forget about spending any more money on expensive face masks at your local beauty supply, supermarket, or department store. Here are eight face masks you can whip up with this simple recipe tutorial.

HONEY FACE MASKS

One of my favorite, all-purpose, ingredients in my home is raw honey. I enjoy it in a morning cup of tea. I drink a warm glass of water with honey to quiet a cough or soothe a sore throat. And of course, you can use it for all-natural skin care.

Honey on Your Face?

It is truly amazing! It can be used as a face wash, just rub 1-2 teaspoons of raw honey on your face and let sit for a minute or two, then rinse with a warm washcloth. Can also be used as a zit zapper, just dab as needed on pimples, then watch them shrivel away to nothing in a matter of only hours. And of course, it can also be used in my personal favorite; facial masks.

Why Honey? You ask.

Raw (unpasteurized) honey is full of great antioxidants which help to fight wrinkles and aging skin. In fact, Cleopatra was a huge fan of honey and used it regularly for her beauty routine. And as everyone knows, she was quite envied and still is for her beautiful, radiant, skin.
Honey is also a natural antibacterial, which helps to prevent and fight acne, a purifier that gently unclogs pores, and a moisturizer which infuses and helps to retain moisture in the skin, leaving your skin feeling soft and supple as nature intended really.

HONEY FACIAL MASK RECIPES

1. Honey and Lavender

Mix one tablespoon of raw honey or Manuka honey (lots of antioxidants for the skin) with 2-3 drops of Lavender essential oil. Apply to face and let sit for 15-20 minutes. Use a warm washcloth to wipe off.

2. Honey and Lemon Facial Mask

Mix one tablespoon of raw honey or Manuka honey with 1-2 drops of Lemon essential oil. Apply to face and let it sit for 15-20 minutes. Use a warm washcloth to wipe off. Be careful to avoid direct sun exposure within 24 hours of using the mask, as lemon oil is photosensitive to the sun.

3. Honey and Yogurt Facial Mask

Mix one tablespoon of raw honey or Manuka honey, 2 tablespoons of plain yogurt. Apply to face and let it sit for 15-20 minutes. Use a warm washcloth to wipe it off.

4. Honey and Patchouli Facial Mask

Mix one tablespoon of raw honey or Manuka honey with 2-3 drops of Patchouli essential oil. Apply to face and let it sit for 15-20 minutes. Use a warm washcloth to wipe off.

5. Honey and Avocado Facial Mask

Mix one tablespoon of raw honey or Manuka honey and 1/2 ripe avocado. Apply to face and let it sit for 15-20 minutes. Use a warm washcloth to wipe off.

6. Honey and Oatmeal Facial Mask

Mix one tablespoon of raw honey or Manuka honey, 2 tablespoons of cooked oatmeal. Apply to face and let it sit for 15-20 minutes. Use a warm washcloth to wipe off.

7. Honey and Uncooked Oatmeal Facial Mask

Mix one tablespoon of raw honey or Manuka honey, 1 tablespoon of uncooked oatmeal (I prefer to grind in a blender to a powder rather than use whole oats for a finer, gentler exfoliation). Apply to face and let it sit for 15-20 minutes. Use a warm washcloth to wipe off.

8. Plain Honey Facial Mask

Want a super, simple facial mask? Just apply 1-2 tablespoons of raw honey or Manuka honey to face and let it sit for 15-20 minutes. Use a warm washcloth to wipe off. It's incredibly moisturizing and balances all skin types.

TONER

There is really so much to be said for the benefits of apple cider vinegar. And for those of you looking for an easy do it yourself completely natural toner, look no further; because I have exactly what you need and have been waiting for right here. After putting together this little brew, I found that I was so in love with it that I will NEVER ever go back to store bought toners with harsh chemicals ever again. Not only is this concoction far more effective, but a large bottle of raw, unfiltered apple cider vinegar usually runs for less than five dollars, and let's just say that there is no reason to argue with that kind of a bargain. Especially, in comparison to what some people are still paying for high end toners which are unsafe and unnatural.

HOW TO MAKE A DIY FACIAL TONER WITH APPLE CIDER VINEGAR

1. For normal to dry skin, mix 1/3 part vinegar to 2/3 part filtered water. Add a few drops, add 5-10 drops per 2 oz. of toner mixture, of Lavender or Frankincense oils.
2. For oily and acne-prone skin, mix 1/2 part vinegar and 1/2 part filtered water. Add a few drops, add 5-10 drops per 2 oz. of toner mixture, of lavender or frankincense oils.

HOW TO STORE DIY FACIAL TONER

Simply store the apple cider facial toner in a glass bottle at room temperature.

HOW TO USE APPLE CIDER FACIAL TONER

Use your homemade DIY facial toner twice a day; first thing in the morning and right before bed.

Can I use Apple Cider Vinegar on my Skin Every day?

Although ACV is acidic, it actually helps to regulate the pH balance of the skin. It's an excellent DIY facial toner and can be used for all skin types. It's also antibacterial and has many anti-inflammatory properties.
For oily and acne-prone skin, ACV helps to treat acne and reduce redness. For dry and normal skin, ACV helps to exfoliate skin and reduce wrinkles.

EYE CREAM

There is really nothing more valuable than a good eye cream. You would be surprised by how much your appearance is boosted, simply by taking the time to use a little bit of this right before going to bed at night. It relieves any puffiness or bags that are caused by stress or the wear and tear of the day. And, it keeps you looking refreshed, regardless of whether or not you slept last night at all.

Ingredients:

1. 1/4 cup green tea
2. 1/4 tsp. citric acid
3. 1 tbsp. rosehip seed oil
4. 1 tbsp. sweet almond oil
5. 1/4 tsp. vitamin E
6. 1 tsp. emulsifying wax
7. 1 drop carrot seed essential Oil
8. 3 drops lavender Essential Oil

Instructions:

1. Brew a cup of green tea.
2. Fill two medium sauce pans about half way full of water.
3. Place a glass bowl with a spout in each pot and turn on stove to medium heat.
4. Add wax, rosehip seed oil, vitamin E oil and sweet almond oil to one pot.
5. Add green tea and citric acid to the other pot.
6. Heat both mixtures until the emulsifying wax has totally melted.
7. Check temperatures of both pots with a thermometer. **BOTH mixtures must be the same temperature before you combine them or your cream won't set.**
8. When both your oil mixture and water mixture reach around 130 degrees, pour your water mixture into your oil mixture.
9. Use a hand held blender and mix your cream.
10. Continue to mix periodically (every 10 minutes or so) until you notice that water is no longer separating on the bottom. This tends to take about 30 minutes to an hour.
11. Once fully mixed, add essential oils then pour into containers.

For those with nut allergies you can use these carrier oils instead, Evening Primrose, Meadowfoam Seed, Apricot Seed, Pomegranate Seed or even Olive Oil.

FACIAL MOISTURIZER 1

Aside from the ACV Toner, I would have to say this is probably one of the easiest do it yourself skin care recipes. Making your own facial moisturizer is really as simple as adding essential oils to a beneficial carrier oil, screwing on the lid, and just using it as needed. I could leave the recipe right there, considering how simple it is. But I will be nice and give you more detailed instructions.

Ingredients

* 2 oz glass dropper bottle
* 2 oz argan oil
* 15 drops Frankincense essential oil
* 10 drops Lavender essential oil

Instructions

1. Add essential oils to the glass dropper
2. Fill Glass Dropper with Argan Oil
3. Screw dropper top on, shake well, and store in a cool, dry, place.
4. Use Morning and Night after each facial wash, or as needed. Approximately 4-6 drops is enough for the entire face.

This recipe will last you about 2-3 months with twice daily use of about 4-6 drops with application.

It is best to use this facial moisturizer in companionship with the other products you made such as the face wash, and the facial toner. Use in succession with the moisturizer coming in last, once in the morning, and once at night before bed for best results.

FACIAL MOISTURIZER 2

MOISTURIZING LOTION

If you are looking for more of a cream like facial moisturizer rather than an oil, here is a recipe that may suit your needs a little better. Plus, it is a bit easier to place in a container and take with you on the go, so you can use it throughout the day as needed. And, not just as a facial moisturizer.

Ingredients:

1. 3 1/2 Tablespoon organic Shea butter
2. 2 Tablespoons Jojoba oil
3. 3 Tablespoons of Aloe Leaf Juice
4. 1 Teaspoon vitamin E oil

5. 4 drops lavender essential oil of choice
6. A pint sized mason jar
7. A small glass jar to store your lotion

Instructions:

1. Add the Shea butter and Jojoba oil to a pint-sized mason jar
2. Place a saucepan on the stove and add a cup of water to it-turn on the heat to medium high
3. Place the mason jar in the saucepan and stir-slowly melting the Shea butter with the jojoba oil.
4. Once the Shea butter and jojoba oil is completely melted, add the aloe juice to the mason jar- (the aloe should be lukewarm)
5. With a hand held immersion blender or food processor -whip the product for at least 5 minutes
6. Add in your essential oil and pour into a small jar
7. Store your face lotion in a sealed glass far and use within 3 months

This WILL NOT work if you swap out the jojoba oil for another type of oil. Jojoba is actually a wax and it is what helps emulsify the aloe water into the rest of the ingredients. Make sure you whip the product well so that the liquid completely blends into jojoba and shea butter.

LIP BALM

I don't know if the rest of you are like me in the sense that you are a bunch of lip balm junkies! I am always carrying around some kind of lip balm, and I make sure that I have back-ups for my backups. There is one in my purse, my bathroom, my gym bag, my car...all the places I don't have lip balm would probably be a shorter list. However, for someone who is such a fiend for a good lip balm, I am quite picky about what I put on my lips. I prefer to steer away from the harsh, nasty chemicals and preservatives found in traditional lip balms. Simply because, the average woman consumes about a pound of cosmetics a year, think about this. You put it on your lips, you eat, you drink, and it goes into your body. So, for many years I believed that buying higher end health food store lip balms was the only way I could go. Until I came across a better and cheaper way to produce my own, for only about twenty-five cents a tube; rather than the usual two to five dollars a tube. Now allow me to blow your mind some more with just how simple this is!

Ingredients

1. 10 drops of lemon or lavender essential oil
2. 1 tbsp organic almond oil
3. 2 tbsp organic extra-virgin coconut oil
4. 1.5 tbsp organic, cosmetic-grade beeswax pastilles
5. Lip balm tubes

Instructions:

1. Use a double boiler on low heat to melt all ingredients (except essential oils).
2. Remove from heat once melted and add essential oils.
3. Fill lip balm tins and let cool for a couple of hours to firm up.

FACIAL SERUM

A simple and very easy recipe for a facial serum that you can make at home, and not have to worry about shelling out a whole lot of money for.

Ingredients

1. 1 oz rosehip seed oil (or other carrier oil but rosehip seed oil is the best for the face)
2. 5 drops Frankincense essential oil
3. 5 drops Myrrh essential oil
4. 5 drops Lavender essential oil
5. 5 drops Aroma Life essential oil blend
6. 2 drops Rose (or Geranium - what I like to call the poor woman's Rose)

Instructions:

1. In a 1 oz glass dropper bottle, add all essential oils. This will be about a 2.5% dilution ratio.
2. Fill the bottle with rosehip seed oil.
3. Use this DIY Facial Serum morning and night around the eyes, mouth and other trouble areas on the face

CHARCOAL PEEL-OFF MASK

If there's one thing I know for sure, that would be the fact that you can waste your money and your time on pore strips that may or may not work, or you can just follow this simple recipe and make enough of this stuff, to where you will never have to buy peel-off mask ever again. Also, if you decide to give it to your friends as gifts, be sure to tell them to break out the camera!

This is so because:

- Activated charcoal absorbs toxins and build-up on the skin, and helps to naturally detoxify.
- Bentonite clay tightens and tones the skin, and draws out impurities deep within the skin.
- Gelatin helps to nourish the skin and helps to act as a binder in this recipe, to draw out impurities. It's the key ingredient that makes this mask peel off.
- Tea Tree Essential Oil clarifies the skin and keeps it clear and smooth.

ABOUT THE MASK

This mask works incredibly well, but you need to know about a few things before you get started:
1. When you apply the mask to your face, make sure you don't apply to the eye brows. The mask is strong and will pull on the eyebrow hairs. Now if you do happen to get on the eyebrows by accident, don't worry. Wipe it off as soon as possible. If it dries and you notice it's in your eyebrows DO NOT PEEL it off. Use a warm washcloth to gently remove the mask.
2. Be sure you also do NOT apply near the eyes. Stay about 2 inches away from the eyes and just above the eyebrow.
3. If at any time when you're peeling the mask off, it hurts or it's just too sensitive to peel, then stop. Use a warm washcloth to gently remove the mask or soak the skin in warm water in the shower and then use a washcloth to remove gently.
4. Peel the mask slowly to draw out the impurities. You'll actually see them on the dried mask areas you peel off.
5. The mask will pull facial hairs too (an added bonus, albeit slightly painful) and the skin will be slightly pink, which is normal with peel-off masks. You might remember this if you've ever used pore strips.

6. Your skin will be as soft and smooth as a baby's butt. Seriously!
7. Discard the dried mask bits in the trash. It won't go down the drain in the sink! Or the toilet!
8. You could just use it on the nose, chin or T-zone if other areas of your face are sensitive.

Ingredients

1. 1 capsule activated charcoal (about 1/4 to 1/3 tsp)
2. 1/4 tsp bentonite clay
3. 1 tsp non-flavored gelatin
4. 1-2 drops tea tree essential oil
5. 2 tsp boiling hot water

Instructions:

1. Remove make up and use a gentle cleanser to clean the face. Pat dry.
2. Open the activated charcoal capsule and add the contents to a small glass or ceramic bowl. Discard the empty capsule.
3. Add bentonite clay and gelatin.
4. Add boiling water and mix well with a mini silicone spatula (avoid metal spoons as the metal may weaken the health properties of the bentonite clay). The gelatin will thicken up the mask.
5. Add 1 drop tea tree oil and mix again.
6. Use a mask brush to apply a layer of the mask to the skin, avoiding eye brows and be careful not to get too close the eyes.
7. Apply mask rather quickly as the mask will continue to thicken up. If the mask in the bowl dries up sooner than you get to apply the mask, add a 1/2 to 1 tsp of boiling hot water again to make the mask liquid again to apply.
8. Once you have a thick layer of the mask on the skin, allow to dry about 20-30 minutes. You may need to wait longer depending on the thickness of the mask. You will feel a slight tingling sensation from the bentonite clay and tea tree oil, both help to remove impurities from the skin.
9. Once the mask is dry, start on an edge (chin or forehead) and slowly peel off the mask until it's completely gone. You can use a warm washcloth to remove any remaining mask on the face.
10. Apply a toner and then follow with a moisturizer to keep the skin nourished.

SHAVE GEL

Here is a little bonus at-home skin care DIY that I found takes things the extra mile, when it comes to being completely conscientious about my skin care. I am telling you to ditch that old shaving cream or shaving gel that is filled with toxic chemicals and God knows what else, and allow me to teach you how to make your own shave gel with these all-natural ingredients instead.

Because of my previous statement, I am sure that you are now aware that the majority of shaving creams and shaving gels which you buy in the store are chock full of harmful chemicals and toxins. All for the sake of making these compounds long lasting in their aerosol containers, without a thought or consideration as to what these compounds will do to a person's skin. The effects are often felt, long after a person has rinsed the gel or cream from their skin. This was not a fact that I even really considered, until I began this journey to rid my home of unnecessary, chemical created and synthetic products. This was the time I decided to take every jar and bottle in my home and educate myself better on what I was actually using, by reading every label I could get my hands on. This was when I also realized just how easy it was to make my own shaving cream or gel at home for myself, and for less than I was paying every couple of weeks for with the drugstore brands. I will show you all how to do this for yourself in just a moment, but first let's take a second to talk about why exactly you need to avoid the shaving products that can be found in the store.

INGREDIENTS TO AVOID IN SHAVE GELS AND SHAVING CREAMS

Go into any store, such as a supermarket, drugstore, or department store and you will most likely see an entire section dedicated solely to shaving cream and shaving gels for both men and women. You will also find that the men's products are priced much lower because the labels use a darker color scheme, even though the contents are made of the same exact products, that serve the same exact function. But because they make the bottles pinker and more appealing, they feel like they can charge us more. Another rant for another day, however, a very valid point, and another reason why you should make your own at home. Even if it is only to not only save yourself some money, but to support that our pricing should not be different just because our genders happen to be.

So when you go into one of these stores, I ask that you venture to turn one of these unequally priced bottles over and read the labels; these are just a few of the ingredients that you will find. And, I think you might even be as disturbed as I was.

RETINYL PALMITATE

This ingredient is composed of palmitic acid and retinol, a byproduct of Vitamin A. Doesn't seem too terribly bad, right? However, data from an FDA study indicates retinyl palmitate, when it is applied to skin, especially when exposed to sunlight, will speed the development of skin tumors and lesions. This ingredient can even be found in some anti-perspirant deodorants. Now you know where all of those little papules come from after you shave your under arms and apply deodorant.

TRIETHANOLAMINE (TEA)

A strong alkaline substance used as a surfactant and pH adjusting chemical. It's known as an immune and respiratory toxicant and allergen.

ISOBUTANE

A hydrocarbon gas, often used as a propellant in aerosolized products, such as hairspray, spray-on deodorant, and fake tanning products; as well as, shave gel and shaving cream. It is a well-known immune and respiratory toxicant and allergen.

METHYLISOTHIAZOLINONE

A commonly used preservative, most popularly associated with allergic reactions. One of the main causes for users being diagnosed with sensitive skin. Also, lab studies on brain cells of mammals have reported that methylisothiazolinone is also a neurotoxin.

PARABENS

This preservative is used to extend the shelf life of many products we use daily. Such as, shave gel, shaving cream, shampoo, conditioner, deodorant, body wash, and several cosmetics. Parabens are a particularly nasty little poison, because they can mimic estrogen and act as potential hormone (endocrine) system disruptors.

FRAGRANCE

Most synthetic fragrances get away with not giving out what they are made of, by labeling their fragrance profiles as proprietary recipes, meaning that the companies are not obligated legally to disclose what they are made of to the public. So, you have no idea what kind of chemical compounds are used to formulate them. Also, meaning that they could be made out of anything really, however toxic, and you will never know. And, many can contain as many as over four thousand different ingredients; that will just be labeled on the packaging simply as "fragrance".

This is just the short list of everything that could be found when researching shave creams, gels, as well as other fragrances and cosmetic products. I found also that the ingredients list can vary quite differently from product to product. But on average, there are usually anywhere from twenty to thirty different ingredients per bottle or can. Again, this does not include or take into consideration the possible four thousand or more ubiquitous ingredients simply labeled "fragrance" which contain even more likely harmful chemicals.
So if you don't know any better, you may very well believe like the rest of the sleeping world, that this is how shaving cream is supposed to be made. It's made to seem like making your own shaving gel or cream is some kind of insurmountable task that requires some twenty to thirty ingredients that would break the bank to acquire, when indeed you could actually accumulate them without getting flagged by some kind of government agency. But I am here to tell you that it is really far simpler than what they would have you believe. A process which only requires four simple ingredients, plus some essential oils or natural fragrances of your choice. Meaning that instead of spending money on something harmful, with obscure ingredients, you can make it at home yourself and know everything that goes into it. Giving you the chance to actually feel secure in the kind of things you are putting on your skin.

HOW TO MAKE THIS SHAVE GEL

Just like the Universe has no concept of difficulty, there should be no difficulty when it comes to making your own at home skin care products. And, this is definitely one of those products that proves this point, because it is really so very easy to make your own DIY Shave Gel. In fact, after the first time, you will see that it only takes a couple of minutes with only a few ingredients: aloe vera gel, fractionated coconut oil, vegetable glycerin, and vitamin E oil.

Essential oils also give this recipe the fragrance, because you are adding your own, you can completely customize the scent profile to your own personal preference. One of my favorite essential oil combinations that works very well for shave gel as well as deodorant, is pine and lavender. Just three drops of each per recipe, is all you will need. If you feel that this scent happens to be a little too masculine for you, then you can try three drops of lavender and three drops of ylang ylang instead, for a more gentle and feminine scent profile.

ABOUT THE INGREDIENTS

Aloe Vera Gel: Aloe Vera is a natural moisturizer and helps to soothe the skin from any kind of outside irritants, as well as burns. It is also very good for keeping the skin hydrated. It also works very well to help to disburse the essential oils evenly through the rest of the product.

Vegetable Glycerin: It helps to keep the Shave Gel well mixed as well as serving as a moisturizer.

Vitamin E Oil: This oil is rich in antioxidants and helps to keep your skin deeply moisturized, as well as helping with the retention of moisture in your skin.

Fractionated Coconut Oil: The reason it is best to use fractionated coconut oil for this recipe rather than just any coconut oil, is because this particular natural compound stays liquid even in colder temperatures. Unlike standard coconut oil. It also helps to moisturize the skin and is great for all types of skin.

Essential Oils: They are used as natural fragrances, and many of them carry healing properties of their own that serve to heal and soothe the skin, as well as helping to boost immunities.

Ingredients:

1. 4 tbsp aloe vera gel

2. 1 tsp fractionated coconut oil

3. 1/2 tsp vegetable glycerin

4. 1/2 vitamin E oil

5. 3 drops Lavender essential oil

6. 3 drops Pine essential oil

Instructions:

In a 2oz bottle or jar, combine all of your ingredients and shake very well.
Apply it to wet skin for a perfectly smooth shave, with lasting moisturizing effects.

RECIPE NOTES

As I stated before, the reason for using fractionated coconut oil rather than standard coconut oil, is because it stays liquid no matter what temperature it is exposed to. So, if you were to use standard coconut oil in this recipe, it will firm up, and will not be easy to spread over your skin. It may even become grainy, which does not feel very pleasant and will not work effectively if you are trying to shave. But just in case you don't happen to have any fractionated coconut oil on hand, you can use sweet almond oil, apricot kernel oil, avocado oil, or even olive oil instead if you need to. Just keep in mind that almond oil and olive oil do have a bit of a scent of their own, and will change the scent profile of your concoction. Also, you need to be sure that all of the carrier oils that you use, are cold pressed organic oils only; as others will have additives and preservatives that will have not only an adverse effect on you, but the mixture as well. So, for a longer lasting mixture that is also good for you, be sure to use only cold pressed organic carrier oils, when you have the occasion to use carrier oils in any of your at-home skin care products.

DEODORANT

I know that home-made deodorant sounds like some kind of hoax you would hear about on social media. Something that you hear about on Pinterest or Instagram and you try it, but it does not quite measure up to what it looked like in the pictures, or have the efficacy that you were aiming for. Some of these other DIY deodorants also often have way too many ingredients that you don't always have on hand, and you feel a little bit like an old timey pharmacist trying to come up with a cure for something. Well, I am here to give you a very simple, four-ingredient only recipe for an at-home deodorant that is not only cheaper, but a healthier alternative to store bought varieties. It is extremely customizable, super inexpensive, and free from all of the disturbing obscure ingredients that can be found in so many of these other products that are advertised to us every day.

This deodorant is only made with three base ingredients, with the option of a fourth being an essential oil for scent and vitality.

These first three staple ingredients are really that in every sense of the word, because they are all things that you can find in your pantry on the daily.

While most deodorants are for the purpose of dealing with body odor, most antiperspirants actually prevent sweat by way of blocking the ducts that produce it. What most people fail to realize is that it is the pheromones in your hair follicles that produce the odor, which is then carried by your sweat, creating a smell. So, if you shave your pits, you are less likely to have any odor, without having to clog your ducts with deodorant. Also, antiperspirants could contain ingredients such as aluminum and artificial fragrances, which can contain up to four thousand different ingredients and they don't have to tell you what they are, as well as triclosan. This ingredient is added to antiperspirant deodorants as a preservative that is supposed to help keep bacteria from growing in the compound, and makes it last longer on the shelf. But what they don't tell you, is that it has highly irritant properties when it comes into contact with skin.

So, my recipe for deodorant does not at all promise to stop you from sweating, but it does work to rid you of any body odor that may secrete from those growing hair follicles. Which is what deodorant is meant to do in the first place, am I right?

Let's get started...

Ingredients:

1. 1/2 cup coconut oil

2. 1/4 cup cornstarch (or arrow root powder if you are currently battling sensitive skin)

3. 1/4 cup baking soda

4. 6 drops Lavender Essential Oil

5. 6 drops Lemongrass Essential Oil

Note: You can use whatever essential oil you choose to create your own custom scent profile, I just chose these because they happen to be my favorites.

Instructions:

The coconut oil is going to be in somewhat of a solid state when you begin, so pop it in the microwave in a microwave safe container for ten seconds at a time, until it is completely melted. Next, mix in your essential oil. Then, add in your dry ingredients, the cornstarch or arrow root powder and baking soda. Mix them until they are completely smooth, no lumps. Finally, transfer the mixture to a jar, and store in a cool, dry place. It may be best to store your deodorant in the refrigerator for a short while, to make sure that the coconut oil goes back to its solid state. You can also clean out and recycle an empty deodorant tube for a mess free application process, if you so desire.

CONCLUSION

The tools and techniques described in this book will be of immense value to you in terms of efficacy and cost savings. You will enjoy making and using every one of them. However, please remember that cosmetics play only a small part in making you look and feel good. To be really healthy and to look your best, your skin care routine must go beyond being skin deep. You must take care of it from the inside as well. You must have good living habits.
You should sleep about eight hours each night, and you must get lots of exercise, sunlight, fresh air and hydration. Proper nutrition is also extremely important for good skin health. Be sure to eat lots of fresh fruit, vegetables, and protein foods, such as lean meat, fish and eggs. Milk is also important.

The simple fact is this; If you take care of yourself, your skin most especially, then you have just gifted yourself one of the best calling cards. No one needs a reason to stand next to a person with healthy, glowing skin. They just find themselves gravitating towards it naturally. It's the first, and instant, visible reflection of what could be on the inside. So, with all this said, I believe you now have absolutely zero excuses to not stay healthy, and look good all your life, because I've introduced you to the alchemy, and it's time for you to get your natural skin magic brewing.

END OF BOOK ONE

OTHER BADCREATIVE BOOKS

The Simple Way To Learn French
The Simple Way To Learn Spanish
The Simple Way To Learn Italian

Thank you for reading, and we hope you'd be kind enough to drop us a review on our amazon page.

www.ingramcontent.com/pod-product-compliance
Lightning Source LLC
Chambersburg PA
CBHW070034040426
42333CB00040B/1674